The Ultimate Red Meat Keto Cookbook

More Than 50 Delicious Ideas for Preparing Red Meat Dishes for the Ketogenic Diet

By

Elisa Hayes

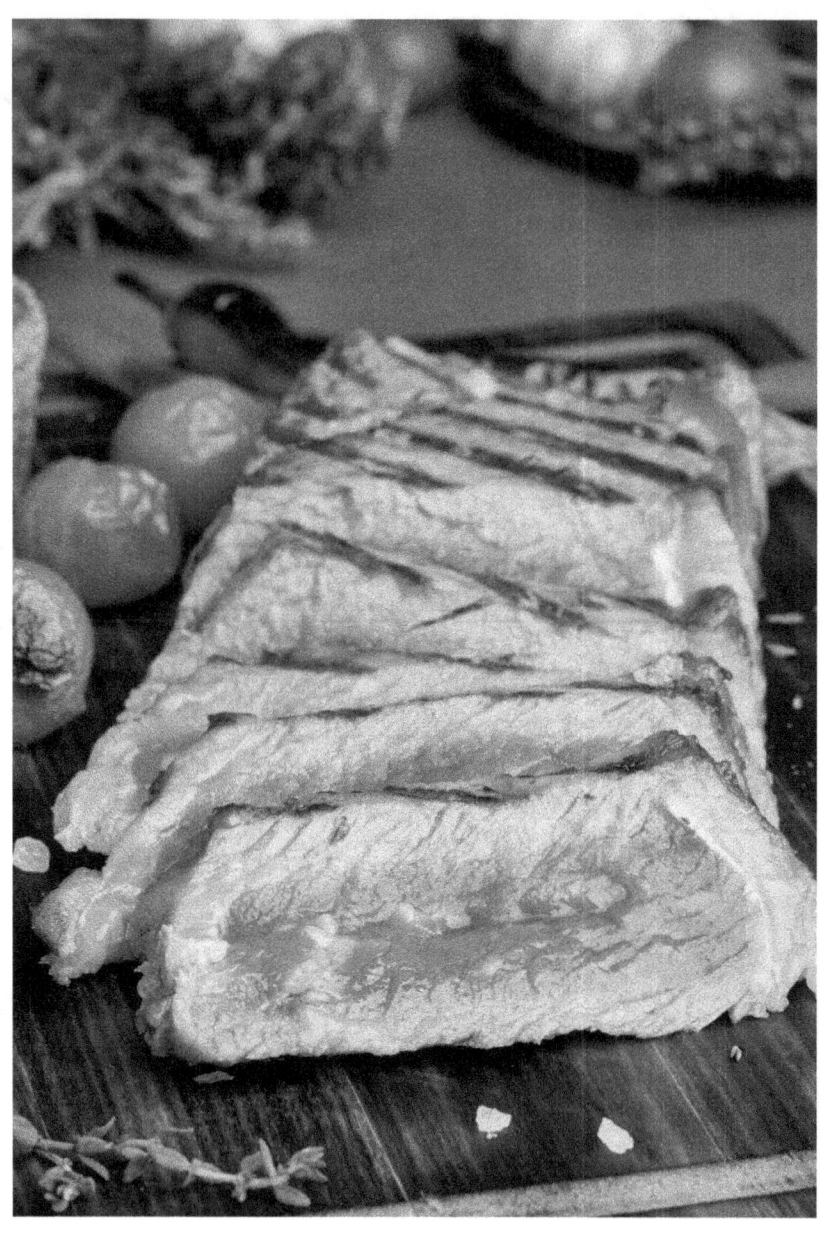

Table of Contents

Introduction — 7
- ALMOND PORK — 11
- CUMIN MEATBALLS — 14
- SWEET PORK — 17
- CURRY MEATBALLS — 18
- THYME PORK CHOPS — 19
- FAJITA PORK — 21
- OREGANO PORK CHOPS — 23
- CHILI PORK SKEWERS — 25
- ROSEMARY PORK TENDERLOIN — 27
- PAPRIKA PORK STRIPS — 29
- JALAPENO PORK CHOPS — 30
- BEEF LASAGNA — 32
- NUTMEG PORK CHOPS — 35
- CHILI GROUND PORK — 36
- THAI STYLE PORK — 37
- 2-MEAT STEW — 40
- PORK AND VEGETABLE MEATBALLS — 42
- SPRING ONION CUBES — 44
- PORK AND MUSHROOMS ROAST — 46
- TURMERIC BEEF TENDERS — 49
- BEEF AND ZUCCHINI MUFFINS — 50
- TOMATO PORK RIBS — 52
- PORK BALLS BAKE — 54
- SAGE PORK CHOPS — 56
- BEEF STUFFED AVOCADO — 57
- TOMATO PULLED PORK — 58
- BEEF WITH PICKLED CHILIES — 61

Almond Meatballs	62
Scallions Beef Meatloaf	64
Bacon Beef	66
Beef Sauce with Broccoli	68
Parsley Taco Beef	70
Meatballs in Coconut Sauce	71
Pork Rolls	74
White Beef Soup	77
Cardamom Sausages	78
Spicy Ground Beef Casserole	79
Marjoram Pork Tenderloin	81
Beef with Noodles	83
Smoked Paprika Pork	86
Sweet Pork Belly	87
Dill Beef Patties	88
Beef Saute	91
Beef and Broccoli Stew	93
Cinnamon Beef Stew	95
Beef and Eggplant Stew	96
Beef Rolls	98
Mint Lamb Chops	100
Chipotle Lamb Ribs	101
Lamb and Pecan Salad	102
Lime Ribs	104

© Copyright 2021 by Elisa Hayes - All rights reserved.

The following Book is reproduced below with the goal of providing information that is as accurate and reliable as possible. Regardless, purchasing this Book can be seen as consent to the fact that both the publisher and the author of this book are in no way experts on the topics discussed within and that any recommendations or suggestions that are made herein are for entertainment purposes only. Professionals should be consulted as needed prior to undertaking any of the action endorsed herein.

This declaration is deemed fair and valid by both the American Bar Association and the Committee of Publishers Association and is legally binding throughout the United States.

Furthermore, the transmission, duplication, or reproduction of any of the following work including specific information will be considered an illegal act irrespective of if it is done electronically or in print. This extends to creating a secondary or tertiary copy of the work or a recorded copy and is only allowed with the express written consent from the Publisher. All additional right reserved.

The information in the following pages is broadly considered a truthful and accurate account of facts and as such, any inattention, use, or misuse of the information in question by the reader will render any resulting actions solely under their purview. There are no scenarios in which the publisher or the original author of this work can be in any fashion deemed liable for any hardship or damages that may befall them after undertaking information described herein.

Additionally, the information in the following pages is intended only for informational purposes and should thus be thought of as universal. As befitting its nature, it is presented without assurance regarding its prolonged validity or interim quality. Trademarks that are mentioned are done without written consent and can in no way be considered an endorsement from the trademark holder.

Introduction

The path to a perfect body and good physical health was very thorny for me. The only one wish which I was making for my birthdays for many years was to be a slim and beautiful girl. Alas, everything can't be as in fairy tales and the miracle didn't happen; my mirror was still showing the same fat, pimple girl. In childhood, the problem of being overweight didn't bother me much; I can say that I didn't care about it at all, I didn't know that weight would be momentous for me. I was an ordinary smiling child, playing with my peers, going to school, and traveling with my parents. That time my chubby cheeks seemed very sweet to everyone. But that was then. At 11-year-old, I went to middle school. New people, new teachers, I had no friends at all. Mentally I was broken. I counted the minutes until the end of the last lesson, to quickly sit in my mom's car and leave school. I started to eat a lot. Now I see that in this way I am stressed, but then the food served as my antidepressant. Dozens of hamburgers, fried potatoes, coke – they were "my best friends". In addition to everything, I started to have horrible skin problems, it seemed to me that there was no place on my face wherever they hadn't appeared yet. Time passed and I no longer loved my reflection in the mirror even in 1%. I couldn't wear the clothes that I liked. I usually wore oversized shorts and t-shirts. I couldn't afford to wear a short dress and high heels. At 15-year-old I weighed more than 270lbs. I remember what I felt in those days, as it is happening now. I felt anger, irritation, hatred, and self-loathing. That prom party was the most terrible day of my life. Thank God it's over!

In those years, the keto diet was not very popular, fasting and drinking diets (which, as you already know, did not help me much) were more popular. Perhaps I wouldn't do anything, but my health problems were becoming more serious. It seemed that my body was simply screaming: please help me!

I remember the day that changed my life on a dime. I came to the clinic with pain in my stomach. But this time, I not only received painkillers but also found a mentor and friend. This was my physician. She had examined me and recommended that I go on a diet. I didn't want to do something and was categorically against it. However, my mind changed when she said: love your body, care about it, and it will thank you. What was my surprise when the diet turned out to be very simple to follow. Is it so easy to love myself? As you could understand I am talking about my favorite keto diet. Every day I was eating a maximum of proteins and a minimum of carbohydrates. That meant to consume meat, poultry, and fish and make restrictions for vegetables, fruits, and sweets. After 2 weeks, I lost 83lbs, and further results were getting better and better. All this time I was under the supervision of a doctor and this yielded results. A year later, I completely changed all the clothes in my wardrobe and oh my God I was able to wear a short dress and skirts! Now I can say that I am the happiest person. It happened because I fell in love with myself and started treating my body as a diamond. My life was filled with bright colors, I have a beloved husband, children, work, friends, I am healthy and like myself in the mirror. I am telling this story to prove that the right diet can solve almost all problems with body and health. It is a fact that our body is capable of dealing with dramatic changes, it is only worth loving it. Never rest on your laurels, never give up and forbid people to say that you cannot do something. You are already a great fellow that you bought this cookbook and decided to take a step ahead in the direction to your dream. Let this book become your ray of hope, a lifesaver on the way to your wonderful transformation. If you believe in yourself and love your body, believe me, the result won't be long in coming. You will see in the mirror a completely new version of yourself, updated physically and mentally! Just trust the keto diet and your inner voice. Set a goal today and start the way of achieving it right now. Don't try to do it all in one time; let it be a small step day by day. Exactly now, this is the right time to start creating a new version of you. If this diet was able to change my life, I'm sure it will help you too!

Almond Pork

Prep time: 10 minutes
Cook time: 20 minutes
Servings: 4

Ingredients:

- ½ cup organic almond milk
- 1-pound pork loin, sliced
- 1 teaspoon ground paprika
- 1 teaspoon ground nutmeg
- 1 tablespoon coconut oil

Method:
1. In the shallow bowl, mix ground paprika and ground nutmeg.
2. Then sprinkle the pork loin with spices and transfer in the skillet.
3. Add coconut oil and roast the pork for 5 minutes per side.
4. After this, add almond milk and carefully mix the meat.
5. Close the lid and cook the pork on medium-low heat for 10 minutes.

Nutritional info per serve: Calories 377, Fat 26.6, Fiber 1, Carbs 2.2, Protein 31.8

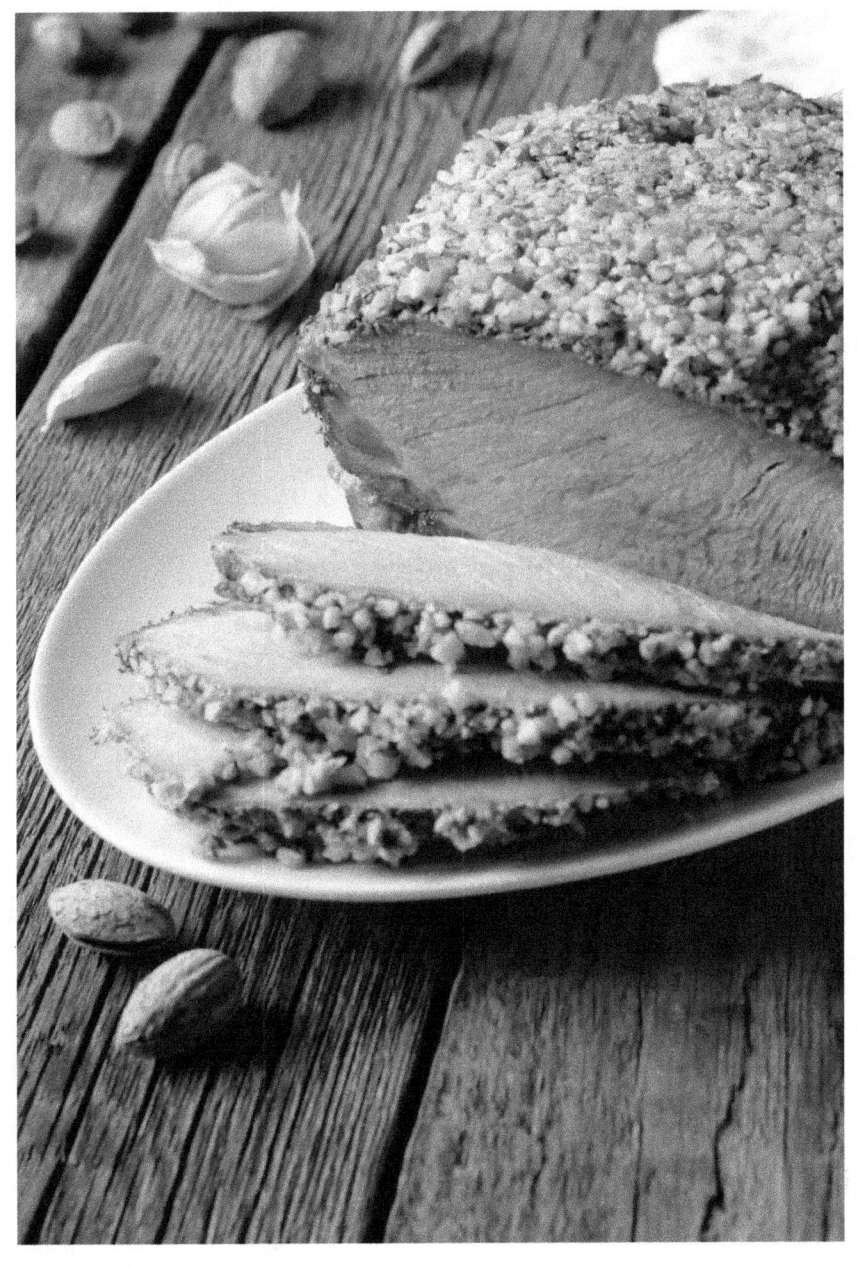

Cumin Meatballs

Prep time: 15 minutes
Cook time: 10 minutes
Servings: 2

Ingredients:

- 1 cup ground beef
- 1 teaspoon ground cumin
- ½ teaspoon chili powder
- 1 teaspoon dried cilantro
- 1 teaspoon minced garlic
- 1 tablespoon olive oil

Method:

1. In the mixing bowl, mix ground beef with ground cumin, chili powder, dried cilantro, and minced garlic.
2. Then make the medium-size meatballs.
3. Preheat the olive oil in the skillet well.
4. Put the meatballs in the hot oil and roast them for 5 minutes per side on the medium heat.

Nutritional info per serve: Calories 198, Fat 15.5, Fiber 0.4, Carbs 1.3, Protein 13.4

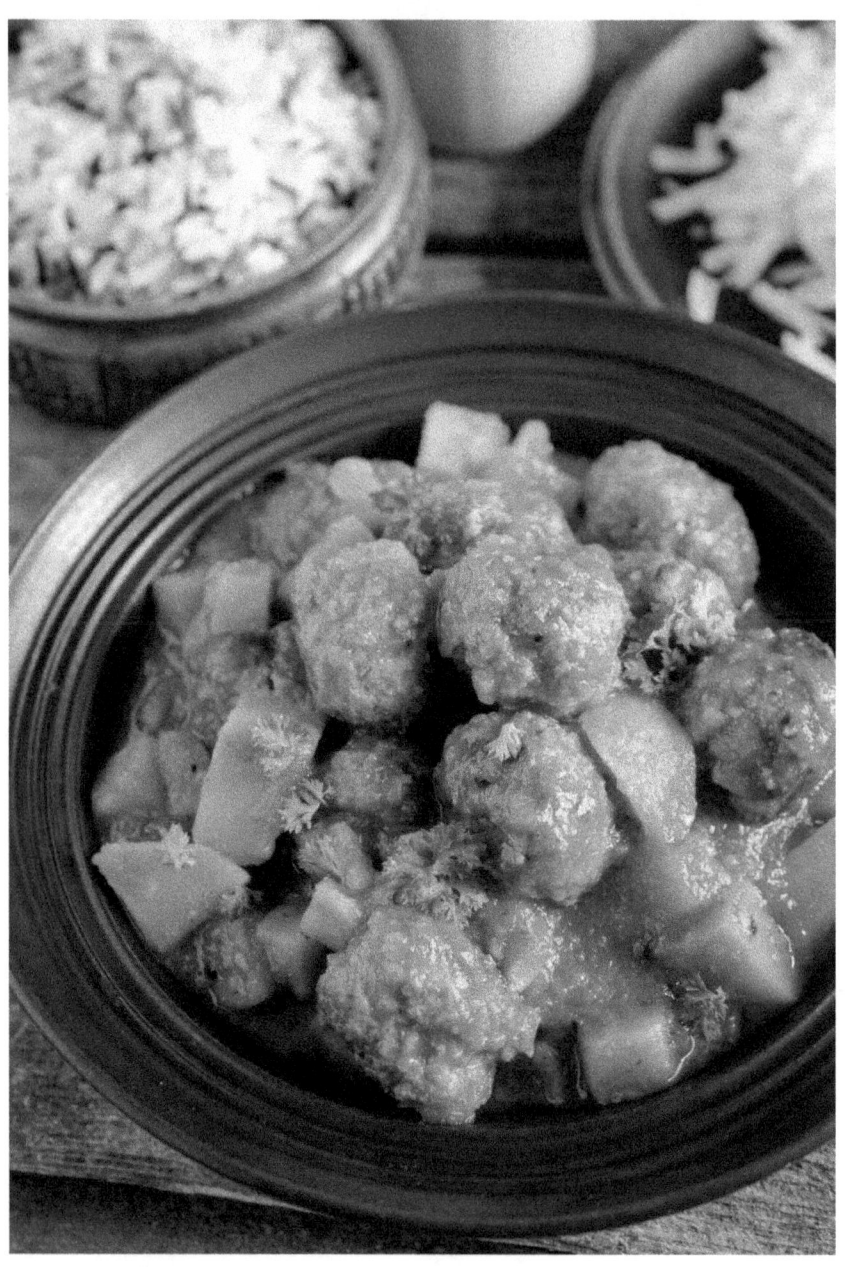

Sweet Pork

Prep time: 10 minutes
Cook time: 20 minutes
Servings: 4

Ingredients:

- 1-pound pork loin, chopped
- 1 tablespoon Erythritol
- 1 tablespoon butter
- 1 teaspoon onion powder
- ½ teaspoon lemon juice

Method:

1. Mix the pork loin with Erythritol, onion powder, and lemon juice.
2. Then melt the butter in the saucepan and add pork.
3. Carefully mix the mixture and roast it for 20 minutes on the medium high heat. Stir the meat from time to time.

Nutritional info per serve: Calories 306, Fat 18.7, Fiber 0, Carbs 2.8, Protein 31.1

Curry Meatballs

Prep time: 15 minutes
Cook time: 10 minutes
Servings:6

Ingredients:

- 2 cups ground pork
- 1 teaspoon curry powder
- 1 teaspoon dried thyme
- 1 tablespoon coconut oil

Method:
1. Mix ground pork with curry powder and dried thyme.
2. Make the meatballs.
3. Then toss the coconut oil in the skillet and preheat it well.
4. Add the meatballs in the hot coconut oil and roast them for 4 minutes per side or until the meatballs are tender and cooked.

Nutritional info per serve: Calories 176, Fat 13.2, Fiber 0.2, Carbs 0.3, Protein 13.5

Thyme Pork Chops

Prep time: 10 minutes
Cook time: 10 minutes
Servings: 4

Ingredients:

- 4 pork chops
- 1 tablespoon dried thyme
- 2 tablespoons olive oil
- 1 teaspoon salt

Method:

1. Rub the pork chops with dried thyme and salt.
2. Then preheat the skillet well, add olive oil and pork chops.
3. Roast the pork chops on medium-high heat for 5 minutes per side.

Nutritional info per serve: Calories 318, Fat 26.9, Fiber 0.3, Carbs 0.4, Protein 18

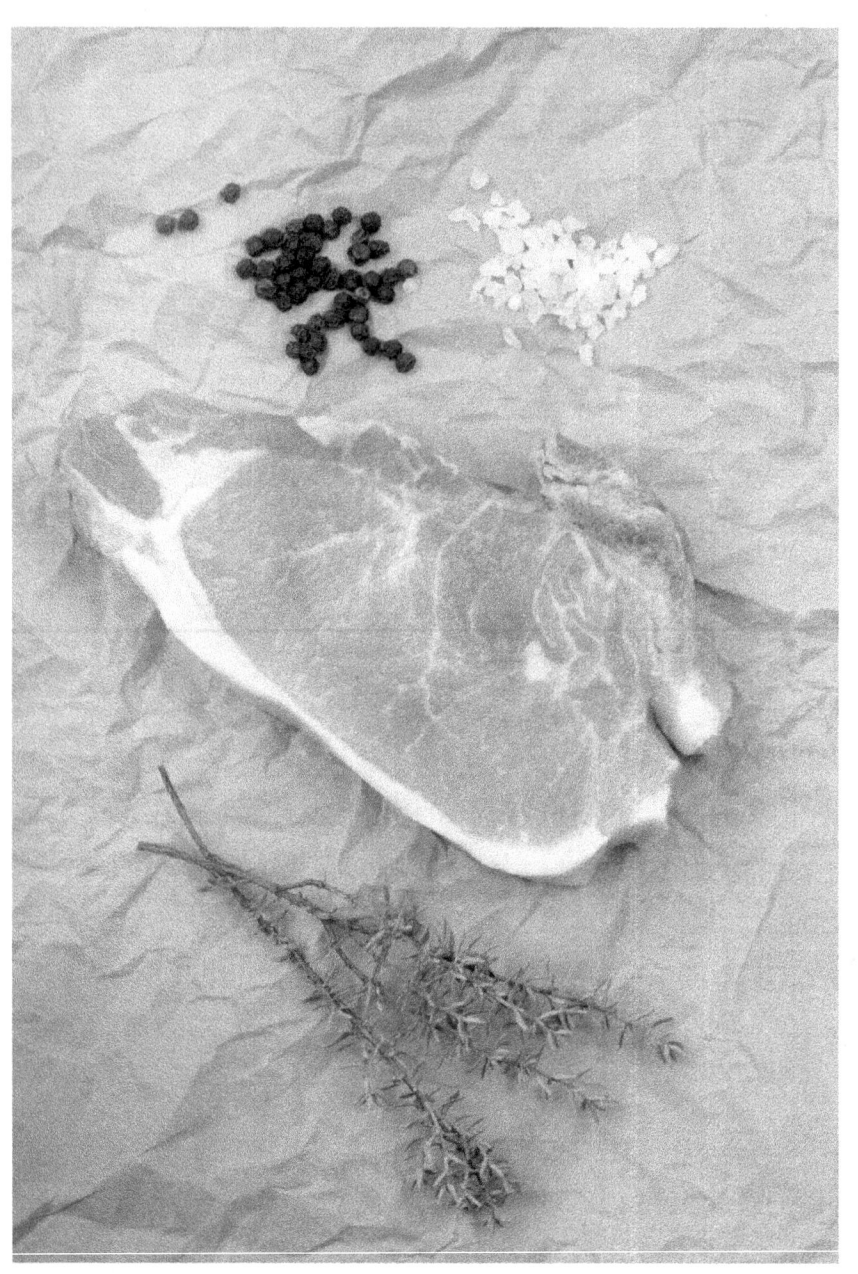

Fajita Pork

Prep time: 10 minutes
Cook time: 20 minutes
Servings: 6

Ingredients:

- 2 cups ground pork
- 1 teaspoon Fajita seasonings
- 2 spring onions, chopped
- 1 tablespoon coconut oil
- ¼ cup of water

Method:

1. Mix the ground pork with Fajita seasonings and chopped onion.
2. Then melt the coconut oil in the saucepan.
3. Add ground pork mixture and roast it for 10 minutes. Stir it from time to time.
4. After this, add water and carefully mix the mixture.
5. Cook the meal on medium heat for 10 minutes more.

Nutritional info per serve: Calories 339, Fat 24, Fiber 0.4, Carbs 2.1, Protein 27

Oregano Pork Chops

Prep time: 10 minutes
Cook time: 30 minutes
Servings: 4

Ingredients:

- 2 tablespoons butter
- 1 tablespoon dried oregano
- 1 tablespoon lemon juice
- 1 tablespoon sesame oil
- 4 pork chops

Method:
1. Brush the baking tray with sesame oil.
2. Then rub the pork chops with dried oregano and sprinkle with lemon juice.
3. Put the pork chops in the prepared baking tray and top them with butter.
4. Bake the pork chops in the oven at 360F for 30 minutes. Flip the pork chops on another side during cooking if needed.

Nutritional info per serve: Calories 341, Fat 29.2, Fiber 0.5, Carbs 0.8, Protein 18.2

Chili Pork Skewers

Prep time: 10 minutes
Cook time: 10 minutes
Servings: 4

Ingredients:

- 1-pound pork loin, cubed
- 1 teaspoon chili powder
- 1 tablespoon sesame oil
- ½ teaspoon ground paprika

Method:
1. Mix the pork cubes with chili powder, ground paprika, and sesame oil.
2. Then string the meat into skewers and grill it at 400F for 5 minutes per side.

Nutritional info per serve: Calories 307, Fat 19.3, Fiber 0.3, Carbs 0.5, Protein 31.1

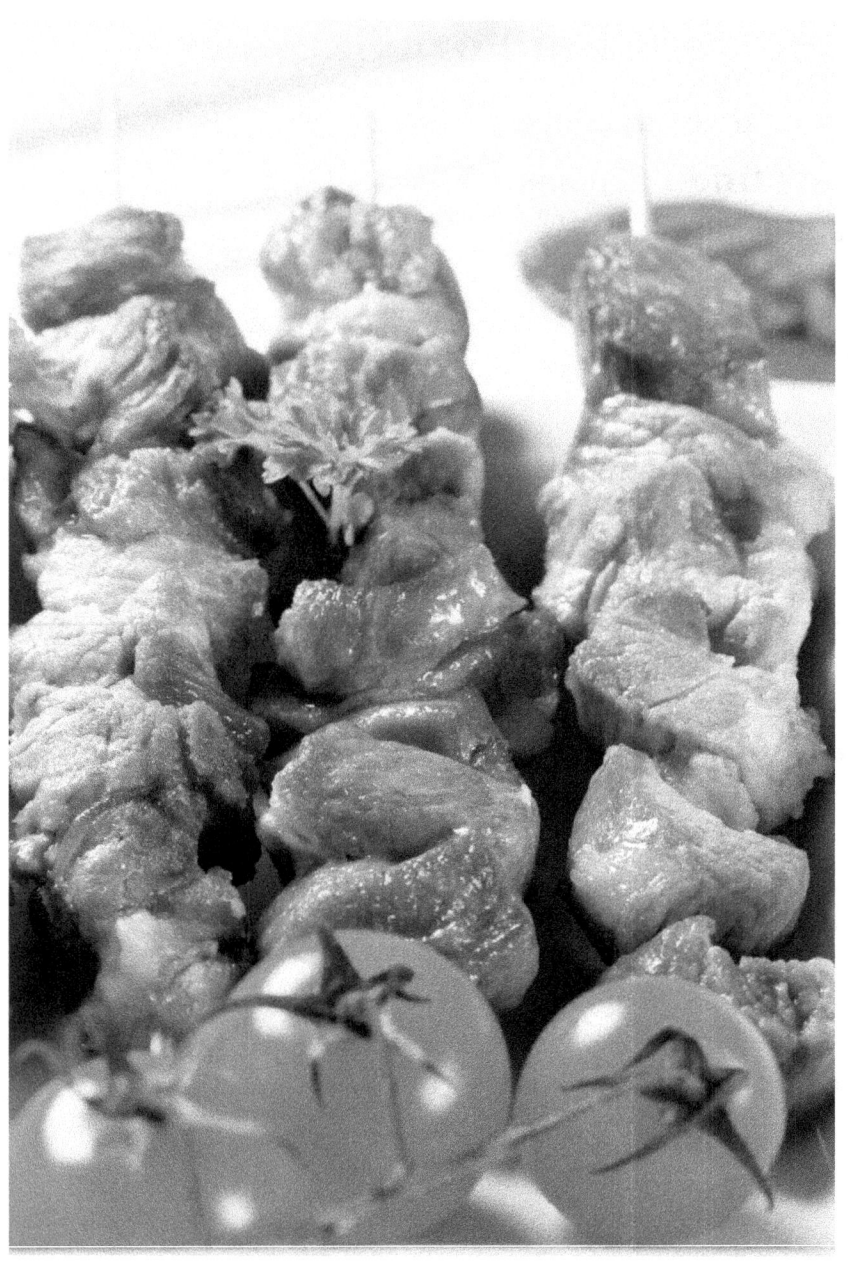

Rosemary Pork Tenderloin

Prep time: 10 minutes
Cook time: 50 minutes
Servings: 4

Ingredients:

- 1-pound pork tenderloin
- 1 teaspoon dried rosemary
- 3 tablespoons butter

Method:
1. Chop the pork tenderloin roughly and put it in the pot.
2. Add dried rosemary and butter.
3. Bake the meat in the preheated 360F oven for 50 minutes.

Nutritional info per serve: Calories 240, Fat 12.7, Fiber 0.1, Carbs 0.2, Protein 29.8

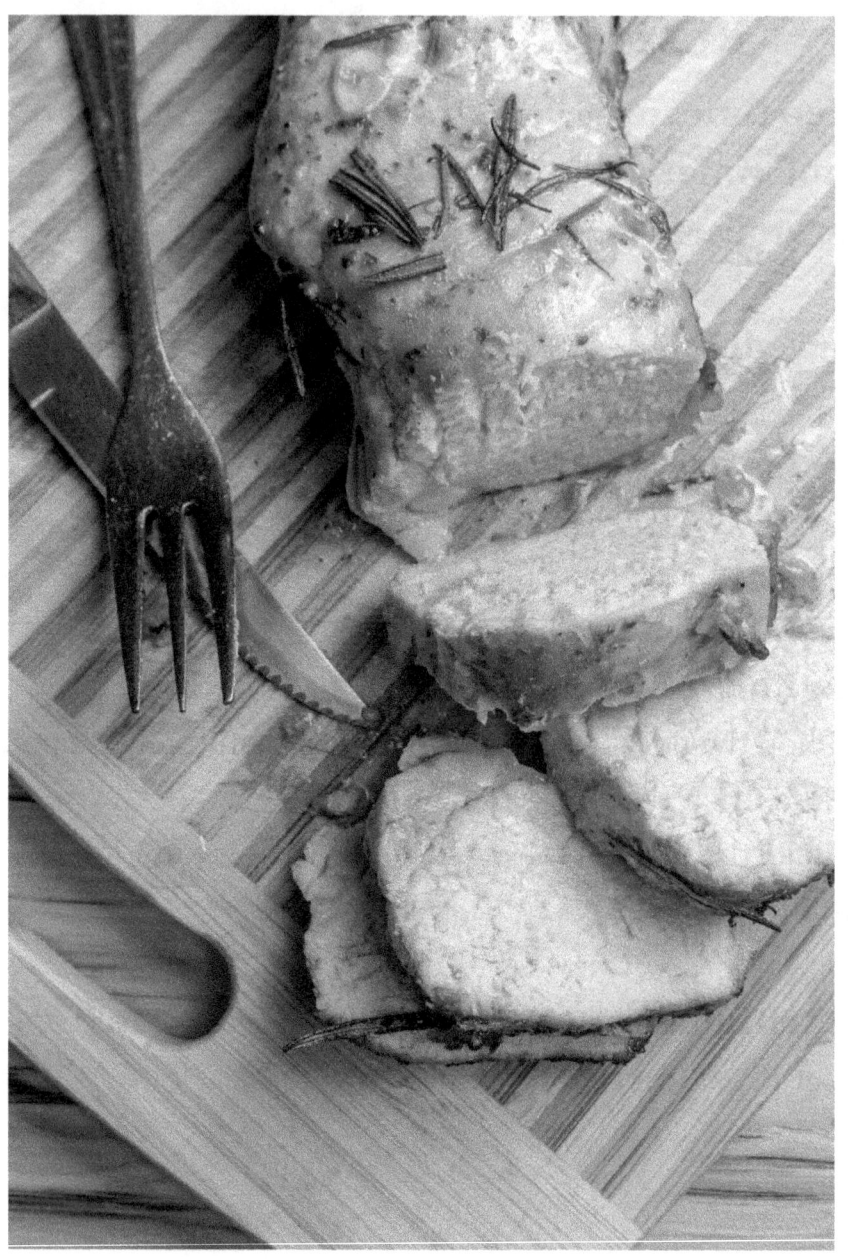

Paprika Pork Strips

Prep time: 10 minutes
Cook time: 20 minutes
Servings: 2

Ingredients:

- 10 oz pork loin, cut into strips
- 1 teaspoon ground paprika
- ½ teaspoon onion powder
- 1 tablespoon sesame oil
- ¼ teaspoon dried oregano

Method:

1. Preheat the sesame oil in the skillet.
2. Add pork loin strips and sprinkle them with ground paprika, onion powder, and dried oregano.
3. Roast the pork strips on medium heat for 15-18 minutes, stir them occasionally.

Nutritional info per serve: Calories 409, Fat 26.7, Fiber 0.5, Carbs 1.2, Protein 39

Jalapeno Pork Chops

Prep time: 10 minutes
Cook time: 35 minutes
Servings: 4

Ingredients:

- 4 pork chops
- 2 jalapenos, sliced
- ½ teaspoon salt
- 2 tablespoons coconut oil
- ½ teaspoon ground black pepper

Method:

1. In the mixing bowl, mix ground black pepper with coconut oil, salt, and sliced jalapeno.
2. Then line the baking tray with baking paper. Put the pork chops inside the tray.
3. After this, top every pork chop with coconut oil mixture.
4. Bake the pork chops in the preheated to 360F oven for 35 minutes.

Nutritional info per serve: Calories 317, Fat 26.7, Fiber 0.3, Carbs 0.6, Protein 18.1

Beef Lasagna

Prep time: 15 minutes
Cook time: 55 minutes
Servings: 6

Ingredients:

- 2 zucchinis, sliced
- 1 cup Cheddar cheese, shredded
- 1 tablespoon keto tomato paste
- 1 cup of water
- 1 teaspoon butter, softened
- 1 teaspoon dried basil
- 2 cups ground beef
- 1 teaspoon chili powder

Method:

1. Grease the casserole mold with butter.
2. Then make the layer from zucchini.
3. Mix ground beef with chili powder and keto tomato paste and put the mixture over the zucchinis.
4. After this, top the ground beef mixture with the layer of zucchinis and sprinkle with cheese and dried basil.

5. Add water and cover the casserole mold with foil.
6. Bake the lasagna at 360F for 55 minutes.

Nutritional info per serve: Calories 182, Fat 12.5, Fiber 1, Carbs 3.2, Protein 14.4

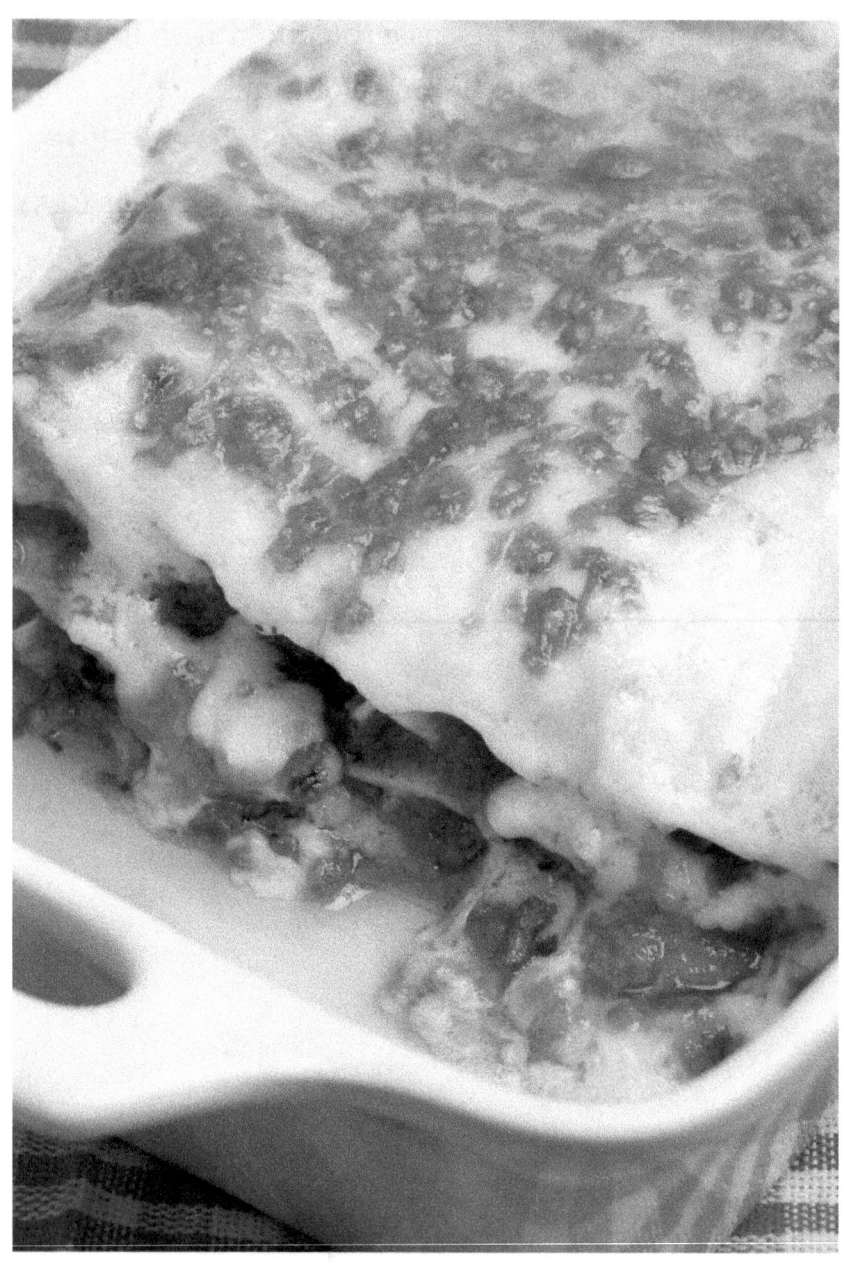

Nutmeg Pork Chops

Prep time: 10 minutes
Cook time: 25 minutes
Servings: 4

Ingredients:

- 4 pork chops
- 1 teaspoon ground nutmeg
- 2 scallions, sliced
- 1 tablespoon coconut oil

Method:
1. Melt the coconut oil in the skillet.
2. Sprinkle the pork chops with ground nutmeg and put in the hot coconut oil.
3. Roast the pork chops for 3 minutes per side.
4. Then add sliced scallions and close the lid.
5. Cook the pork chops for 15 minutes on the medium-low heat.

Nutritional info per serve: Calories 299, Fat 23.5, Fiber 0.7, Carbs 2.8, Protein 18.3

Chili Ground Pork

Prep time: 10 minutes
Cook time: 25 minutes
Servings: 2

Ingredients:

- 1 cup ground pork
- 1 chili pepper, chopped
- 1 tablespoon sesame oil
- ½ teaspoon keto tomato paste
- ¼ cup of water

Method:
1. Pour the sesame oil in the saucepan and preheat it well.
2. Add ground pork and chili pepper. Roast the meat for 5 minutes on the medium heat.
3. Then add keto tomato paste and water. Carefully mix the mixture and close the lid.
4. Simmer the meal on medium heat for 15 minutes.

Nutritional info per serve: Calories 527, Fat 39.3, Fiber 0.1, Carbs 0.4, Protein 40.3

Thai Style Pork

Prep time: 10 minutes
Cook time: 25 minutes
Servings: 6

Ingredients:

- 1-pound pork loin, sliced
- 1 teaspoon curry powder
- 1 teaspoon cayenne pepper
- 1 teaspoon chili flakes
- 2 tablespoons butter
- ¼ cup of water

Method:

1. Melt the butter in the saucepan.
2. Add sliced pork loin. Sprinkle the meat with curry powder, cayenne pepper, and chili flakes. Carefully mix the meat and cook it for 10 minutes.
3. Then add water and carefully mix the mixture.
4. Close the lid and cook the pork on medium heat for 10 minutes.

Nutritional info per serve: Calories 219, Fat 14.5, Fiber 0.2, Carbs 0.4, Protein 20.8

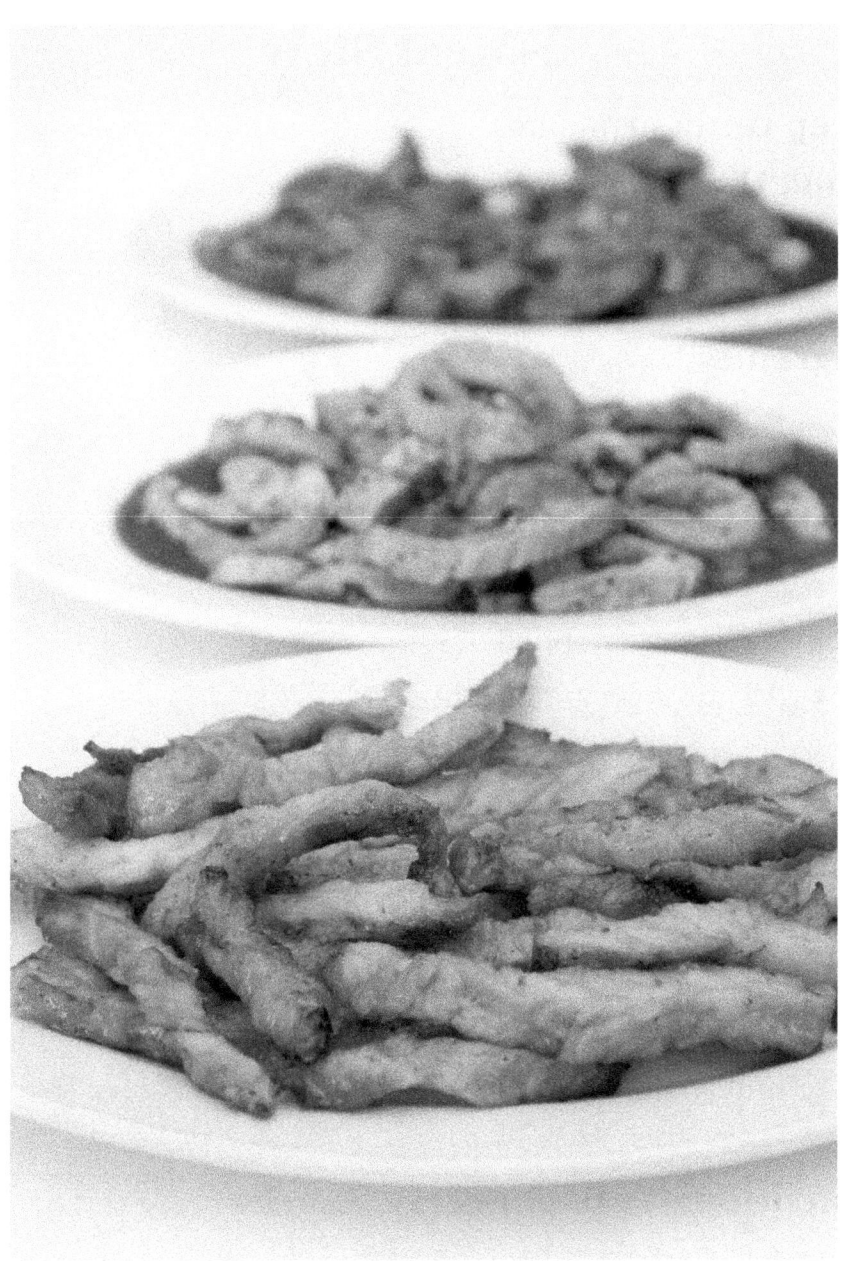

2-Meat Stew

Prep time: 10 minutes
Cook time: 50 minutes
Servings: 3

Ingredients:

- 7 oz beef sirloin, chopped
- 4 oz pork tenderloin, chopped
- 4 cups of water
- 2 oz leek, chopped
- ½ cup celery stalk, chopped
- 1 teaspoon keto tomato paste
- 1 teaspoon dried thyme

Method:

1. Put all ingredients in the saucepan and carefully mix.
2. Close the lid and cook the stew on medium-low heat for 50 minutes.

Nutritional info per serve: Calories 194, Fat 5.6, Fiber 0.8, Carbs 3.7, Protein 30.5

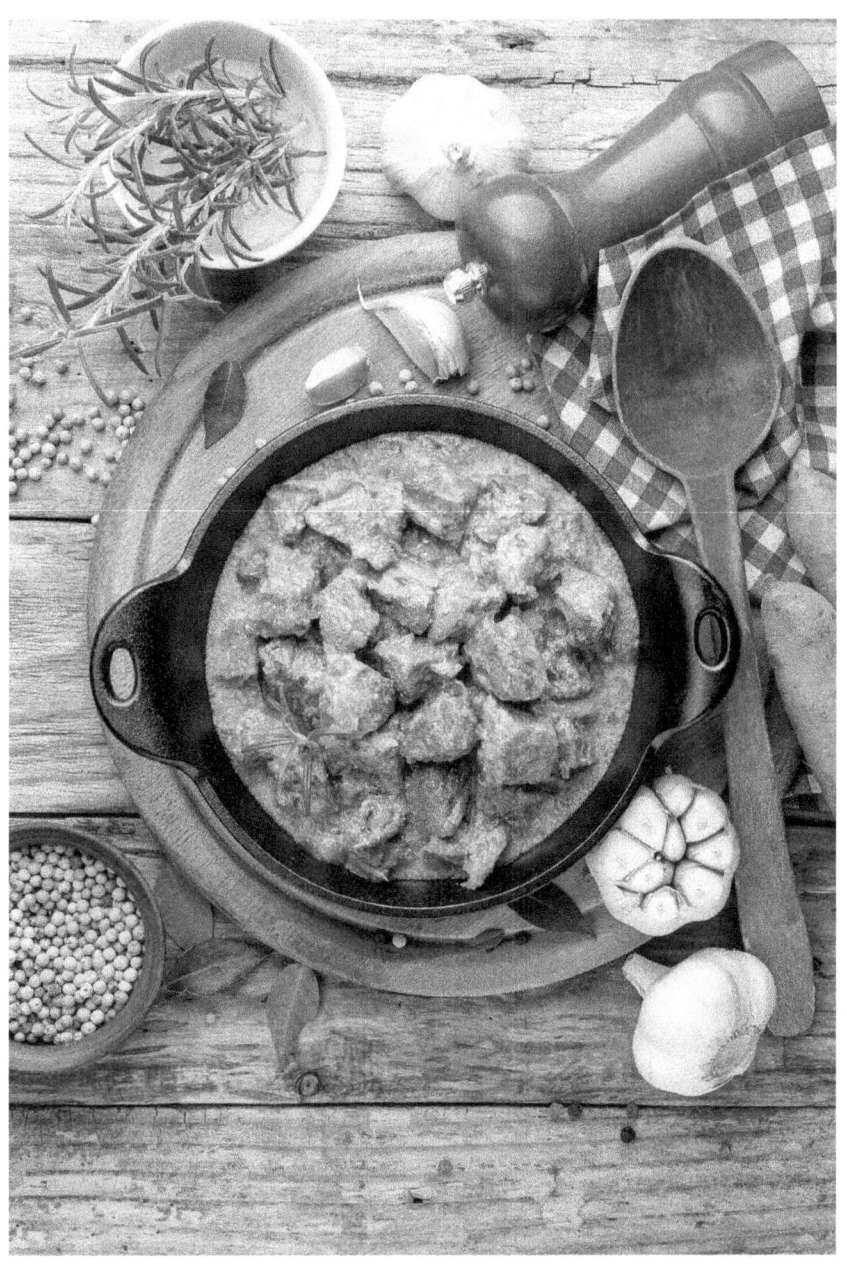

Pork and Vegetable Meatballs

Prep time: 10 minutes
Cook time: 25 minutes
Servings: 6

Ingredients:

- ½ cup cauliflower, shredded
- 2 cups ground pork
- 1 tablespoon almond flour
- 1 egg, beaten
- 1 teaspoon dried basil
- 1 teaspoon onion powder

Method:
1. In the mixing bowl, mix shredded cauliflower with ground pork, and almond flour.
2. Then add egg, dried basil, and onion powder.
3. Make the small meatballs from the meat mixture.
4. Line the baking tray with baking paper.
5. Put the meatballs in the tray and bake them at 360F for 25 minutes or until the meatballs are light brown.

Nutritional info per serve: Calories 351, Fat 24.7, Fiber 0.7, Carbs 1.8, Protein 28.9

Spring Onion Cubes

Prep time: 10 minutes
Cook time: 25 minutes
Servings: 4

Ingredients:

- 1-pound pork loin, cubed
- 3 spring onions, diced
- 1 tablespoon coconut oil
- 1 teaspoon cayenne pepper
- 1 teaspoon salt

Method:
1. Mix the pork loin cubes with cayenne pepper and salt.
2. Then melt the coconut oil in the saucepan.
3. Add pork loin cubes and roast them for 5 minutes per side.
4. Add diced spring onion and carefully mix the meat mixture.
5. Cook the meal on medium-low heat for 10 minutes more.

Nutritional info per serve: Calories 316, Fat 19.3, Fiber 0.7, Carbs 2.8, Protein 31.3

Pork and Mushrooms Roast

Prep time: 10 minutes
Cook time: 30 minutes
Servings: 6

Ingredients:

- 3½ pounds beef roast, chopped
- 1 cup mushrooms, chopped
- 1 teaspoon ground coriander
- 1 teaspoon ground nutmeg
- ½ teaspoon salt
- 2 tablespoons coconut oil

Method:
1. Grease the baking tray with coconut oil.
2. Then mix beef roast with ground coriander, ground nutmeg, and salt.
3. Put the meat in the baking tray and add mushrooms.
4. Bake the mixture in the preheated to 360F oven for 30 minutes. Stir the mixture from time to time to avoid burning.

Nutritional info per serve: Calories 535, Fat 21.2, Fiber 0.2, Carbs 0.6, Protein 80.7

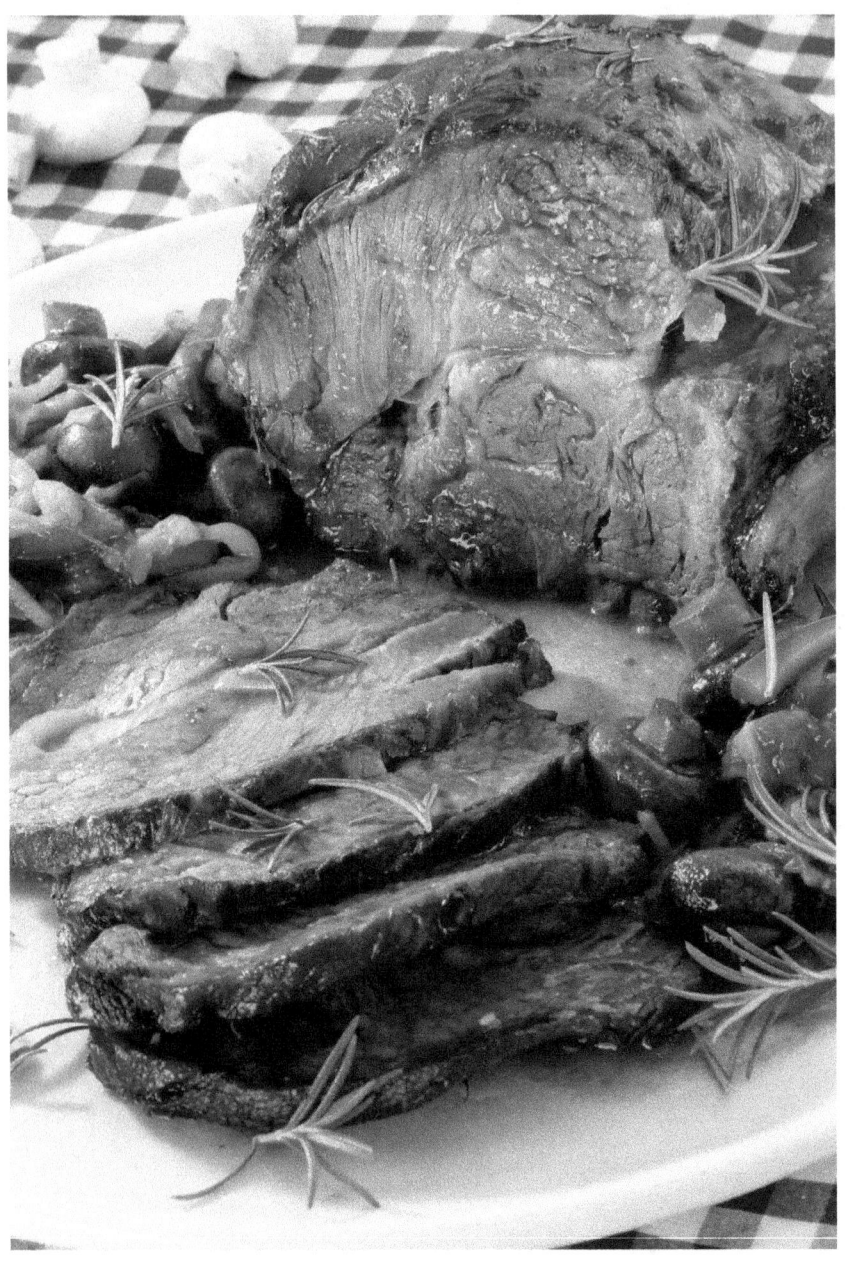

Turmeric Beef Tenders

Prep time: 10 minutes
Cook time: 25 minutes
Servings: 4

Ingredients:

- 1-pound beef tenderloin, cut into tenders
- 1 teaspoon ground turmeric
- 1 tablespoon apple cider vinegar
- 1 teaspoon keto tomato paste
- 2 tablespoons coconut oil

Method:

1. Melt the coconut oil in the skillet.
2. Then put the meat in the hot oil and sprinkle it with ground turmeric, apple cider vinegar, and keto tomato paste.
3. Carefully mix the mixture and roast it on medium-low heat for 20 minutes.

Nutritional info per serve: Calories 296, Fat 17.2, Fiber 0.2, Carbs 0.6, Protein 32.9

Beef and Zucchini Muffins

Prep time: 10 minutes
Cook time: 25 minutes
Servings: 4

Ingredients:

- ½ cup zucchini, grated
- 1 cup ground beef
- 1 teaspoon ground black pepper
- 1 teaspoon garlic powder
- 1 tablespoon coconut flour
- 1 teaspoon salt
- 1 egg, beaten

Method:

1. In the mixing bowl, mix grated zucchini with ground beef, ground black pepper, garlic powder, salt, coconut flour, and egg.
2. After this, transfer the mixture in the muffin molds.
3. Bake the muffins for 25 minutes at 355F.

Nutritional info per serve: Calories 87, Fat 5.3, Fiber 0.4, Carbs 1.5, Protein 8.3

Tomato Pork Ribs

Prep time: 20 minutes
Cook time: 35 minutes
Servings: 6

Ingredients:

- 2-pound pork ribs, roughly chopped
- 1 tablespoon keto tomato paste
- 1 teaspoon cayenne pepper
- 3 tablespoons lemon juice
- 1 tablespoon avocado oil

Method:

1. In the mixing bowl, mix avocado oil with lemon juice, cayenne pepper, and keto tomato paste.
2. Then coat the pork ribs in the tomato mixture and leave for 10-15 minutes to marinate.
3. Roast the pork ribs in the preheated to 365F oven for 35 minutes. Flip the ribs on another side halfway of cooking.

Nutritional info per serve: Calories 421, Fat 27.2, Fiber 0.3, Carbs 1, Protein 40.3

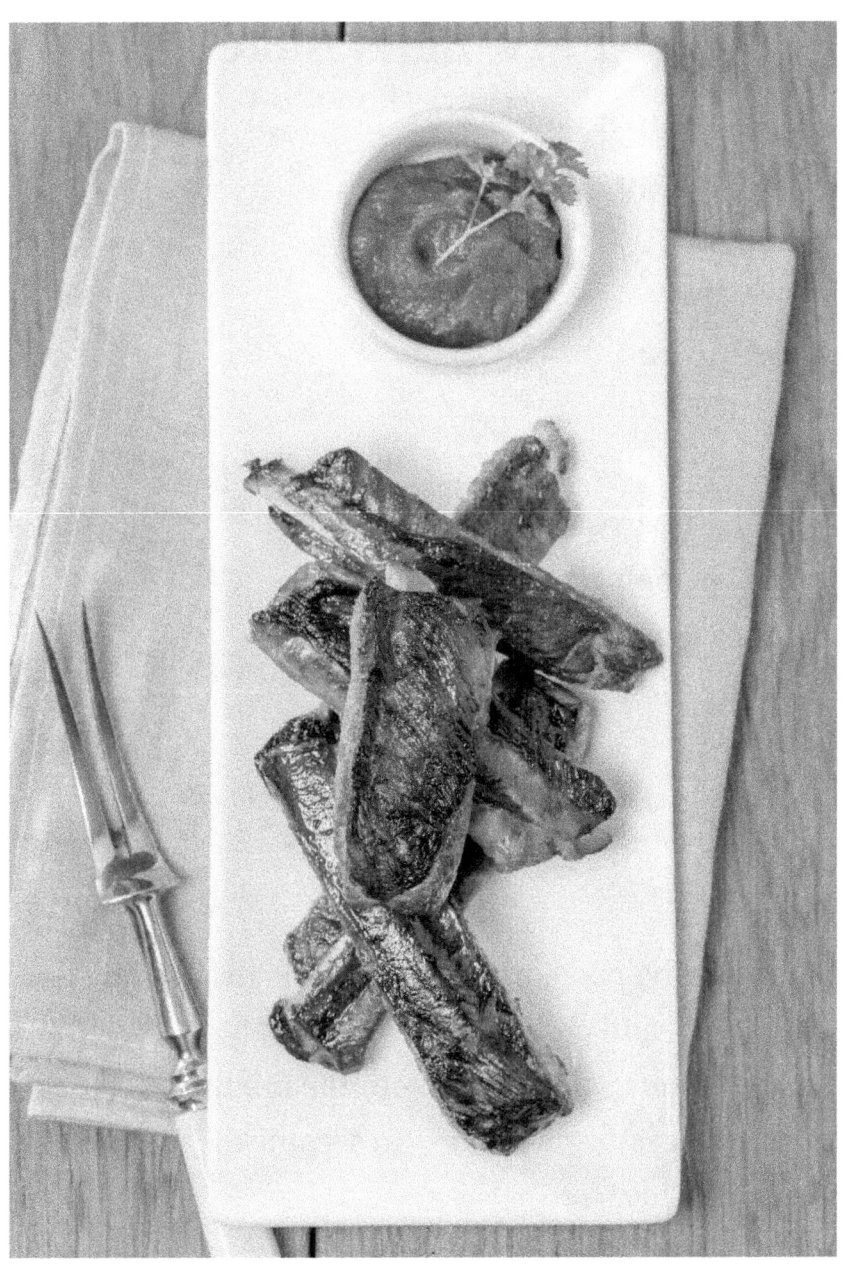

Pork Balls Bake

Prep time: 10 minutes
Cook time: 40 minutes
Servings: 8

Ingredients:

- 2 cups ground pork
- 1 teaspoon dried basil
- 1 teaspoon ground black pepper
- 1 teaspoon chili powder
- 1 cup Mozzarella, shredded
- ½ cup of coconut milk
- 1 teaspoon sesame oil

Method:

1. In the mixing bowl, mix ground pork, dried basil, ground black pepper, and chili powder.
2. Make the small meatballs from the mixture.
3. Brush the casserole mold with sesame oil and put the meatballs inside.
4. Add coconut milk and Mozzarella.
5. Bake the meal for 40 minutes at 355F.

Nutritional info per serve: Calories 284, Fat 21.1, Fiber 0.5, Carbs 1.3, Protein 21.5

Sage Pork Chops

Prep time: 10 minutes
Cook time: 15 minutes
Servings: 7

Ingredients:

- 7 pork chops
- 1 tablespoon dried sage
- ½ teaspoon salt
- 2 tablespoons coconut oil, melted

Method:
1. Rub the pork chops with dried sage and salt.
2. Then melt the coconut oil in the skillet.
3. Put the pork chops inside and cook them for 6 minutes per side.

Nutritional info per serve: Calories 290, Fat 23.8, Fiber 0.1, Carbs 0.2, Protein 18

Beef Stuffed Avocado

Prep time: 15 minutes
Cook time: 0 minutes
Servings: 2

Ingredients:

- 7 oz beef loin, boiled, shredded
- 1 teaspoon plain yogurt
- 1 garlic clove, diced
- 1 avocado, halved, pitted
- 1 pecan, chopped

Method:
1. Scoop ½ part of all avocado flesh and mash it.
2. Then mix mashed avocado flesh with pecan, garlic, and plain yogurt. Add shredded beef loin.
3. Fill the avocado halves with beef mixture.

Nutritional info per serve: Calories 438, Fat 32.9, Fiber 7.5, Carbs 10.3, Protein 29.5

Tomato Pulled Pork

Prep time: 15 minutes
Cook time: 50 minutes
Servings: 4

Ingredients:

- 1-pound pork shoulder
- 4 cups of water
- 1 teaspoon peppercorn
- 1 teaspoon cayenne pepper
- 1 tablespoon keto tomato paste

Method:

1. Mix water with pork shoulder and bring the mixture to boil. Add peppercorn, and cayenne pepper. Simmer it for 45 minutes.
2. After this, remove the pork shoulder from the liquid and shred it.
3. Mix the shredded pork with ½ part of the remaining liquid and keto tomato paste. Bring the mixture to boil and carefully mix.

Nutritional info per serve: Calories 337, Fat 24.4, Fiber 0.4, Carbs 1.4, Protein 26.7

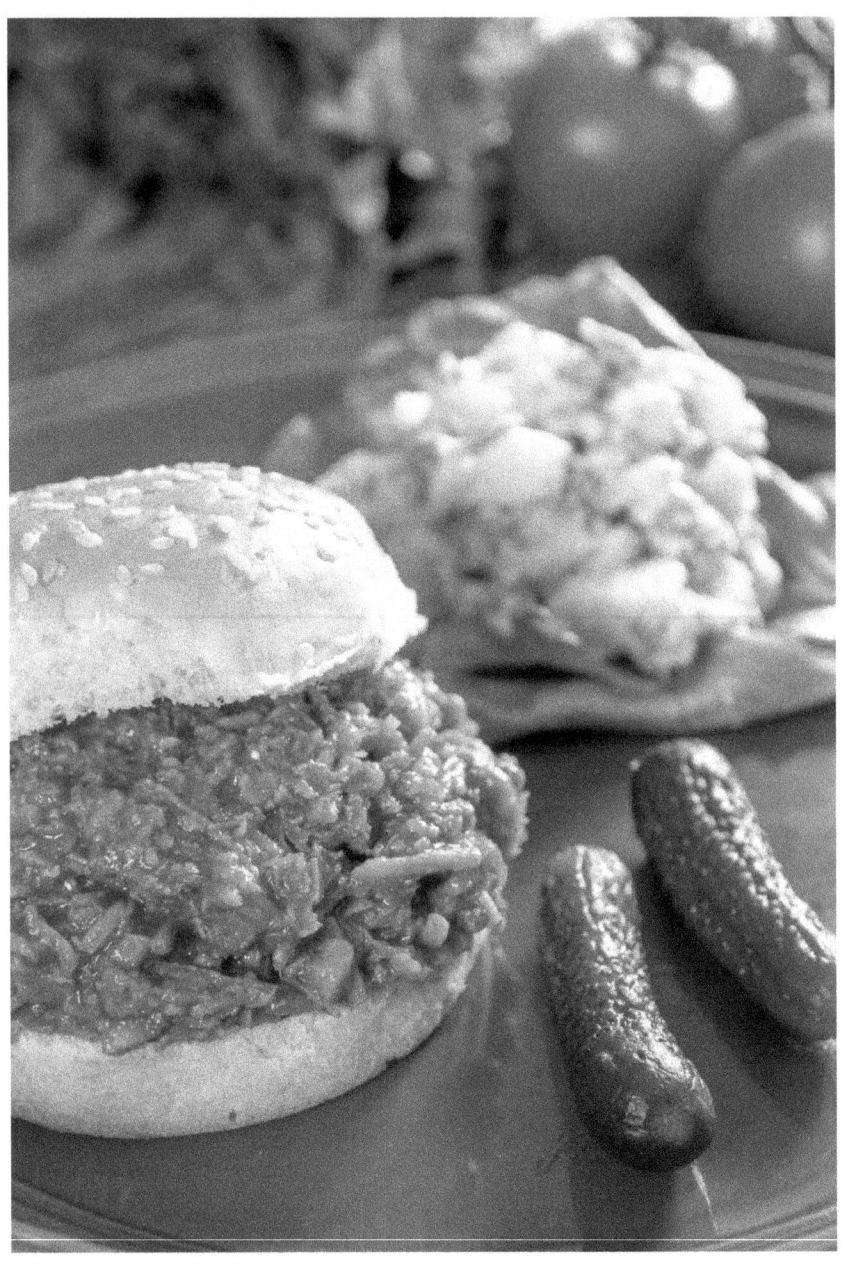

Beef with Pickled Chilies

Prep time: 10 minutes
Cook time: 20 minutes
Servings: 4

Ingredients:

- 2 oz chilies, chopped, pickled
- 1 jalapeno, chopped
- 1-pound beef loin, sliced
- 1 tablespoon coconut oil
- 1 teaspoon ground paprika

Method:

1. Toss the coconut oil in the skillet.
2. Add sliced beef loin and roast it for 2 minutes per side.
3. Then sprinkle the meat with ground paprika, jalapeno, and chilies.
4. Carefully mix the meal and cook it for 15 minutes on medium heat. Stir it from time to time.

Nutritional info per serve: Calories 284, Fat 13.8, Fiber 4.4, Carbs 10.4, Protein 32

Almond Meatballs

Prep time: 15 minutes
Cook time: 15 minutes
Servings: 4

Ingredients:

- 1 cup ground beef
- 1 tablespoon almond flour
- 1 oz almonds, grinded
- 1 oz Parmesan, grated
- 1 tablespoon coconut oil

Method:

1. Mix ground beef with almond flour, almonds, and grated cheese.
2. Make the meatballs from the meat mixture.
3. Preheat the coconut oil well.
4. Put the meatballs in the hot oil and roast them for 4 minutes per side on medium heat.

Nutritional info per serve: Calories 182, Fat 15, Fiber 1.6, Carbs 3.3, Protein 10.5

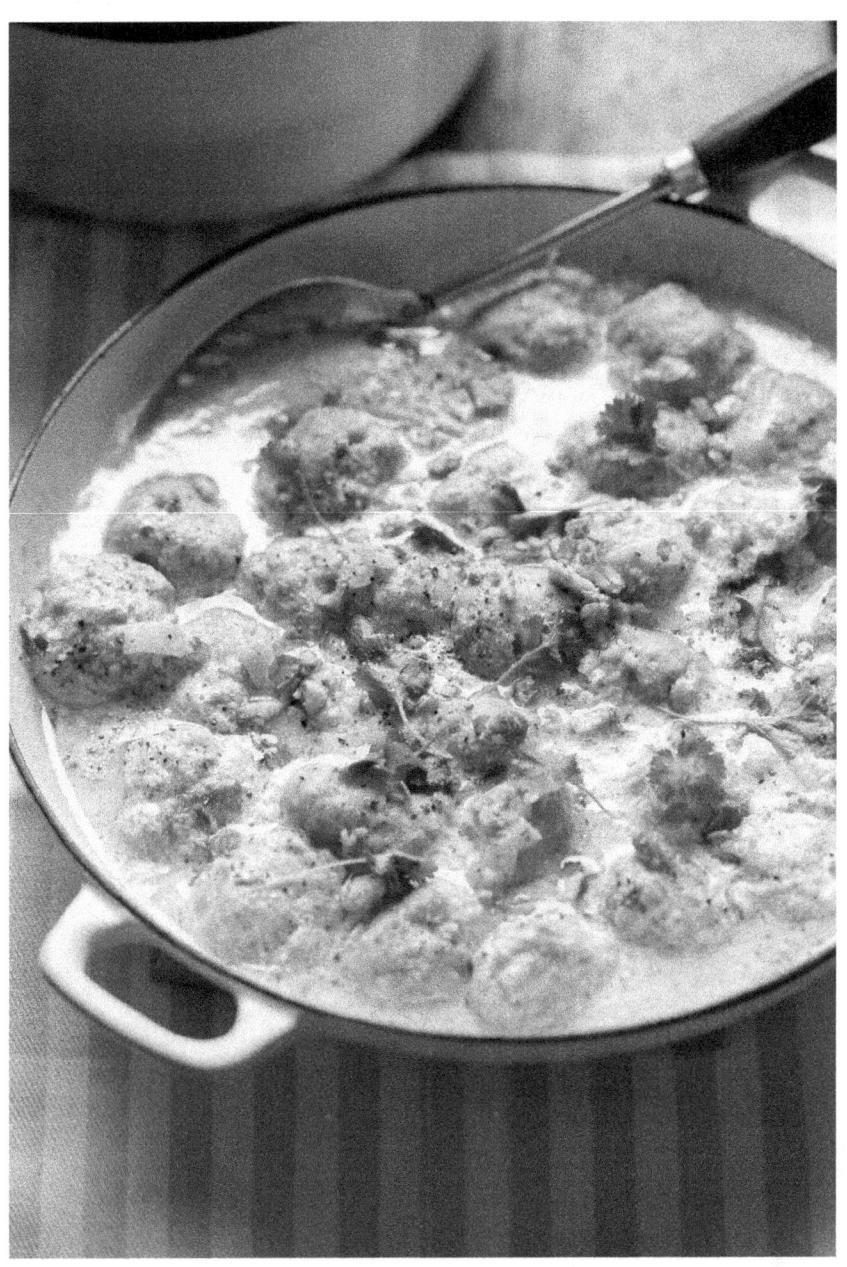

Scallions Beef Meatloaf

Prep time: 10 minutes
Cook time: 50 minutes
Servings: 6

Ingredients:

- 2 oz scallions, diced
- 1 egg, beaten
- 1 teaspoon salt
- 1 teaspoon dried basil
- 2 cups ground beef
- 1 teaspoon butter, softened

Method:
1. Grease the loaf mold with butter from inside.
2. Then mix all remaining ingredients in the mixing bowl.
3. Transfer the mixture in the loaf mold and flatten well.
4. Bake the meatloaf for 50 minutes at 360F.

Nutritional info per serve: Calories 89, Fat 5.4, Fiber 0.4, Carbs 1.8, Protein 8.1

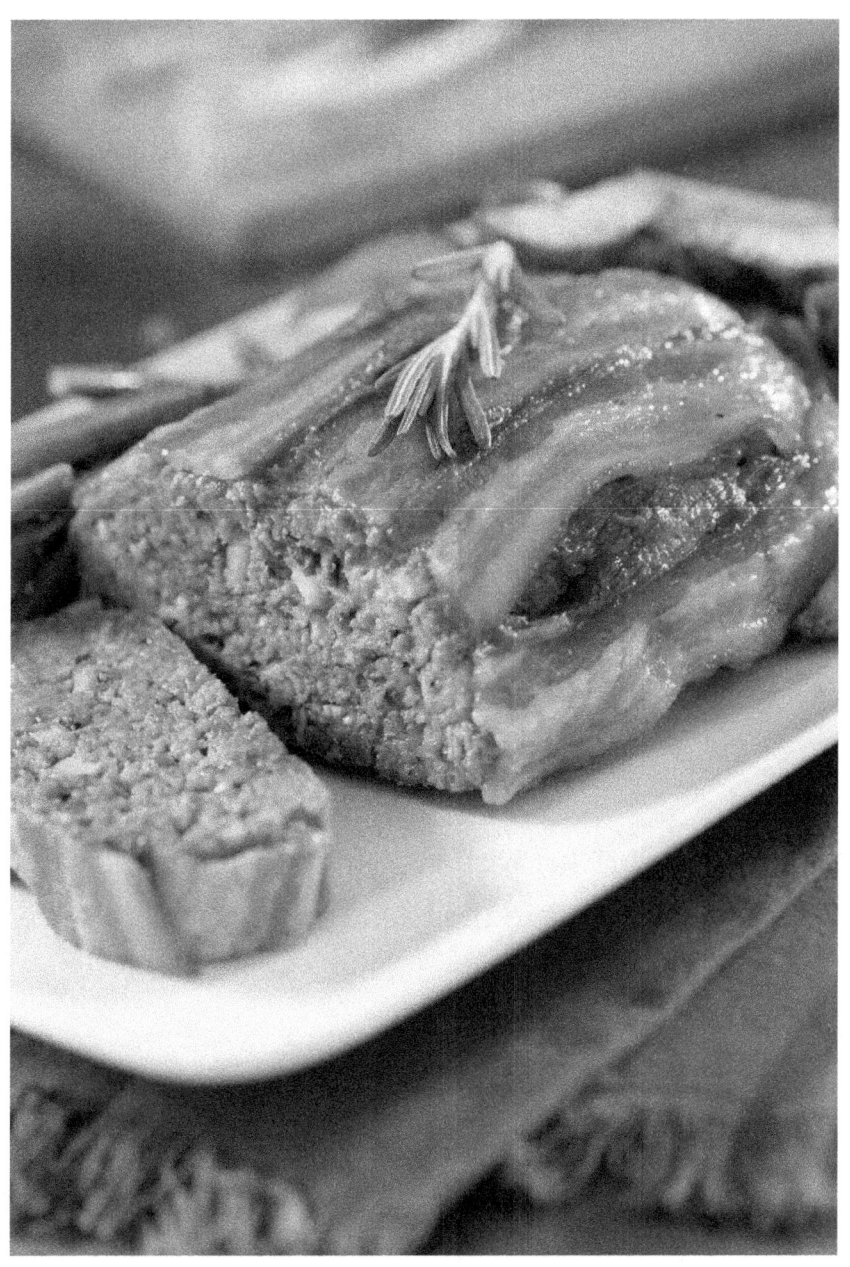

Bacon Beef

Prep time: 15 minutes
Cook time: 55 minutes
Servings: 4

Ingredients:

- 1-pound beef brisket
- 2 oz bacon, sliced
- 1 teaspoon ground cardamom
- 1 tablespoon olive oil
- 1 teaspoon salt

Method:

1. Rub the beef brisket with ground cardamom and salt.
2. Then wrap the beef in the bacon and brush with olive oil.
3. Wrap the meat in the foil and bake at 360F for 55 minutes.

Nutritional info per serve: Calories 134, Fat 8.1, Fiber 0.6, Carbs 2.7, Protein 12.2

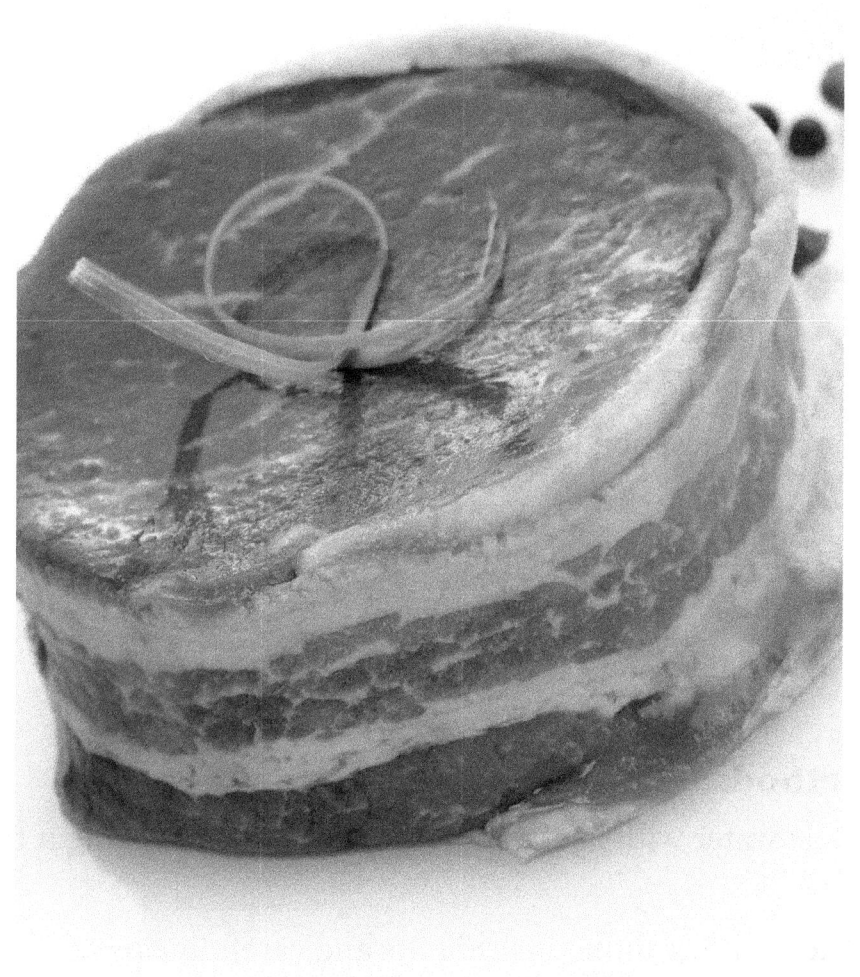

Beef Sauce with Broccoli

Prep time: 10 minutes
Cook time: 35 minutes
Servings: 6

Ingredients:

- 1 cup broccoli, shredded
- 1-pound beef loin, diced
- 2 spring onions, diced
- 1 tablespoon keto tomato paste
- 2 cups of water
- 1 tablespoon coconut flour
- 1 teaspoon salt
- ½ teaspoon cayenne pepper

Method:

1. Mix water with beef loin in the saucepan and bring it to boil.
2. Add all remaining ingredients and carefully mix until homogeneous.
3. Simmer the meal on medium heat for 25 minutes.

Nutritional info per serve: Calories 163, Fat 6.8, Fiber 1.8, Carbs 4.6, Protein 21.3

Parsley Taco Beef

Prep time: 10 minutes
Cook time: 15 minutes
Servings: 4

Ingredients:

- 1 teaspoon taco seasonings
- 1 teaspoon dried parsley
- 1-pound beef loin
- 1 tablespoon coconut oil

Method:
1. Chop the beef loin and mix it with parsley and taco seasonings.
2. Then put the meat in the hot skillet.
3. Add coconut oil and roast it for 15 minutes on medium heat. Stir the meat every 3 minutes during cooking.

Nutritional info per serve: Calories 238, Fat 12.9, Fiber 0, Carbs 0.5, Protein 30.3

Meatballs in Coconut Sauce

Prep time: 10 minutes
Cook time: 15 minutes
Servings: 6

Ingredients:

- 2 cups ground beef
- 1 teaspoon dried cilantro
- 1 teaspoon chili powder
- 1 teaspoon minced garlic
- 1 cup coconut cream
- 1 teaspoon ground turmeric
- 1 teaspoon ground coriander
- 1 tablespoon butter

Method:
1. Mix ground beef with all ingredients except butter and coconut cream.
2. Make the meatballs.
3. Melt the butter in the saucepan.
4. Add meatballs and roast them for 3 minutes per side on medium heat.

5. Then add coconut cream and close the lid.
6. Simmer the meatballs on medium heat for 10 minutes.

Nutritional info per serve: Calories 178, Fat 15.6, Fiber 1.1, Carbs 2.9, Protein 8.1

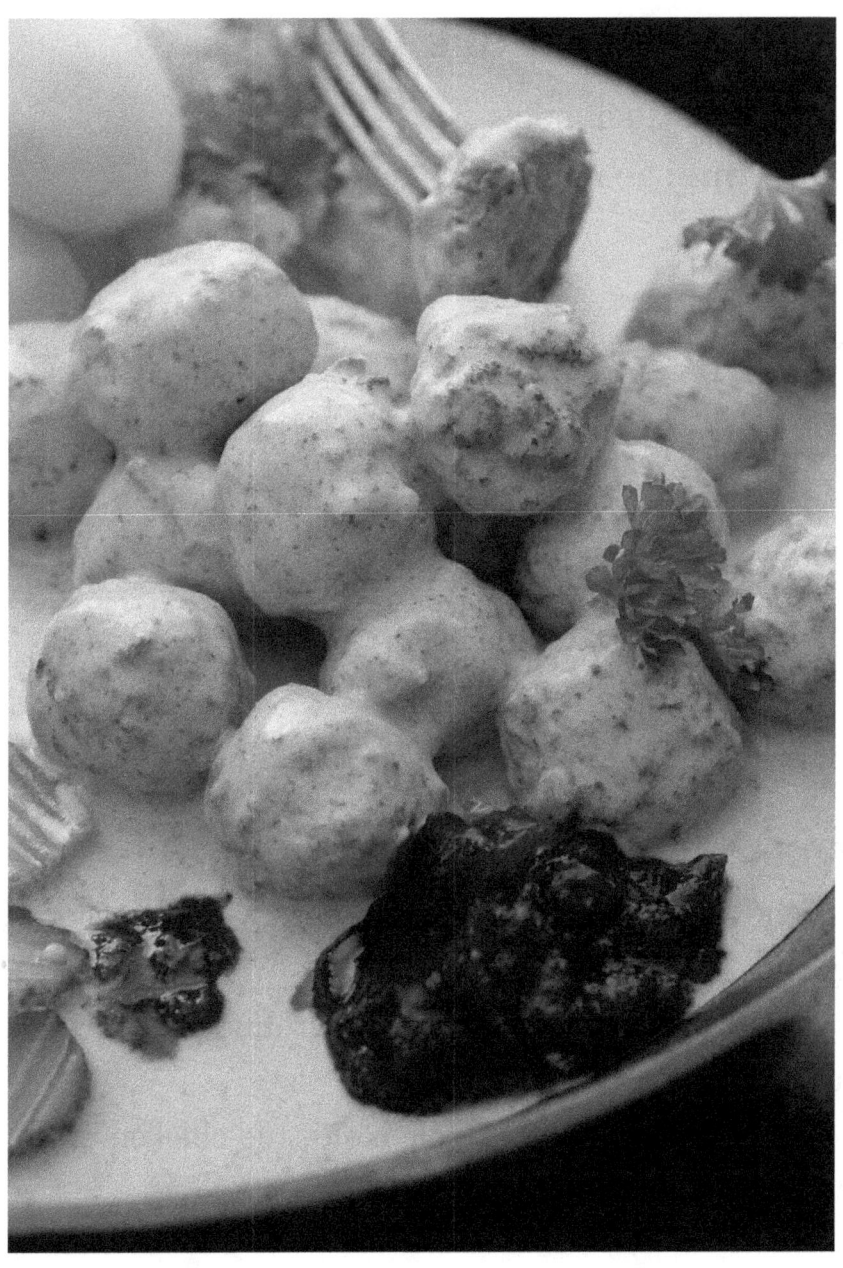

Pork Rolls

Prep time: 10 minutes
Cook time: 30 minutes
Servings: 4

Ingredients:

- 4 white cabbage leaves
- 1 cup ground pork
- 1 garlic clove, diced
- 1 teaspoon cayenne pepper
- 1 cup chicken broth
- 1 teaspoon dried dill

Method:

1. In the mixing bowl, mix ground pork with diced garlic, cayenne pepper, and dried dill.
2. Then fill the cabbage leaves with ground pork mixture and roll them.
3. Put the rolls in the casserole mold, add chicken broth, and bake at 360F for 30 minutes.

Nutritional info per serve: Calories 74, Fat 4.5, Fiber 0.6, Carbs 1.7, Protein 6.6

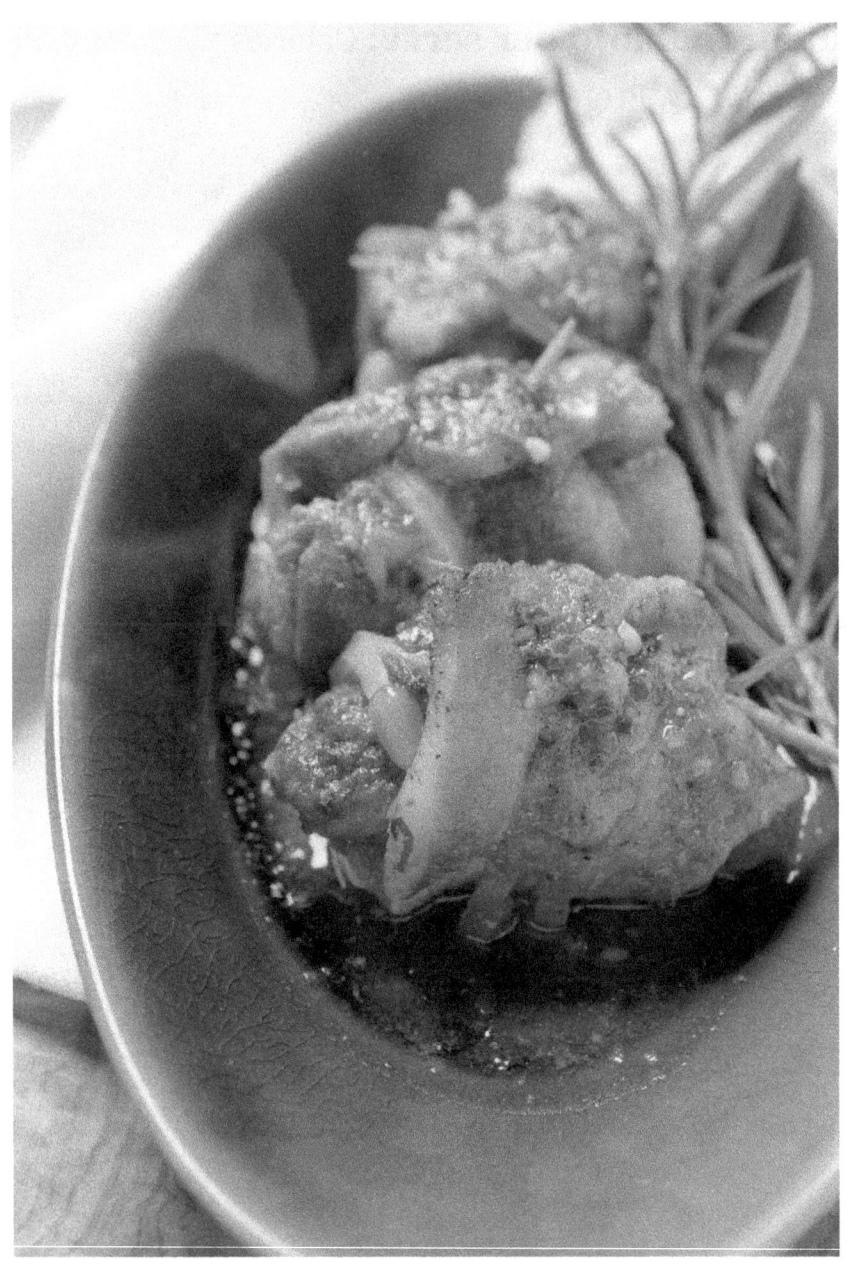

White Beef Soup

Prep time: 10 minutes
Cook time: 30 minutes
Servings: 8

Ingredients:

- 1 cup of coconut milk
- ½ cup fresh parsley, chopped
- 1-pound beef loin, chopped
- ½ cup celery stalk, chopped
- 1 teaspoon salt
- 1 teaspoon white pepper

Method:

1. Put all ingredients in the saucepan and stir well.
2. Simmer the soup on medium-high heat for 30 minutes.

Nutritional info per serve: Calories 156, Fat 11.3, Fiber 1, Carbs 2.9, Protein 11.3

Cardamom Sausages

Prep time: 10 minutes
Cook time: 15 minutes
Servings: 4

Ingredients:

- 1-pound pork sausages
- 1 teaspoon ground cardamom
- 1 teaspoon sesame oil
- 1 tablespoon plain yogurt

Method:
1. Mix pork sausages with plain yogurt and ground cardamom.
2. Then preheat the skillet well. Add sesame oil.
3. Add the pork sausages and roast them for 6 minutes per side.

Nutritional info per serve: Calories 399, Fat 33.4, Fiber 0.1, Carbs 0.6, Protein 22.3

Spicy Ground Beef Casserole

Prep time: 10 minutes
Cook time: 40 minutes
Servings: 6

Ingredients:

- 1 cup Mozzarella, shredded
- 1 cup ground beef
- 1 teaspoon Cajun seasonings
- 1 teaspoon sesame oil
- 1 cup asparagus, chopped
- ½ cup chicken broth

Method:

1. Brush the casserole mold with sesame oil.
2. Then mix ground beef with Cajun seasonings. Put the meat mixture in the casserole mold and flatten it gently.
3. Then top the meat with asparagus and shredded Mozzarella.
4. Add chicken broth.
5. Cook the casserole in the preheated to 360F oven for 40 minutes.

Nutritional info per serve: Calories 61, Fat 3.7, Fiber 0.5, Carbs 1.1, Protein 5.7

Marjoram Pork Tenderloin

Prep time: 10 minutes
Cook time: 40 minutes
Servings: 4

Ingredients:

- 1-pound pork tenderloin
- 1 teaspoon dried marjoram
- 1 teaspoon ground coriander
- 1 tablespoon coconut oil
- 2 tablespoons apple cider vinegar

Method:

1. Mix ground coriander with dried marjoram.
2. Then rub the pork tenderloin with the spice mixture and sprinkle with apple cider vinegar.
3. Grease the baking pan with coconut oil and put the pork tenderloin inside.
4. Cook the meat at 360F for 40 minutes in the oven.

Nutritional info per serve: Calories 193, Fat 7.4, Fiber 0.1, Carbs 0.2, Protein 29.7

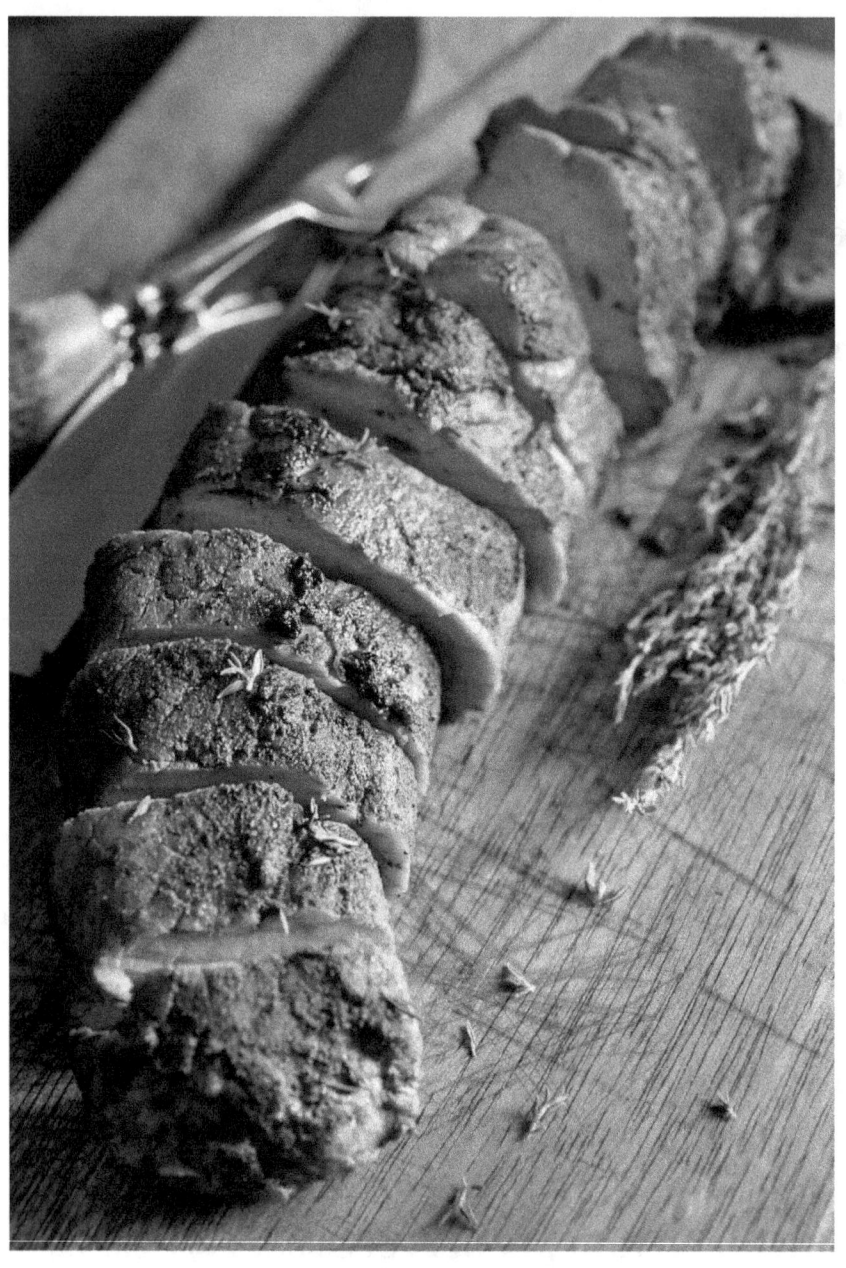

Beef with Noodles

Prep time: 10 minutes
Cook time: 20 minutes
Servings: 5

Ingredients:

- 9 oz ground beef
- 1 teaspoon keto tomato paste
- 1 teaspoon ground turmeric
- 1 teaspoon ground paprika
- 1 tablespoon butter
- ½ cup of coconut milk
- 2 zucchinis, spiralized

Method:

1. Toss butter in the saucepan and melt it.
2. Add ground beef, turmeric, and paprika. Stir the mixture and cook it for 10 minutes.
3. Then mix it carefully and add keto tomato paste and coconut milk. Simmer the mixture for 5 minutes.
4. Add spiralized zucchinis and cook the meal for 3 minutes on medium heat.

Nutritional info per serve: Calories 187, Fat 11.4, Fiber 1.7, Carbs 4.7, Protein 17.1

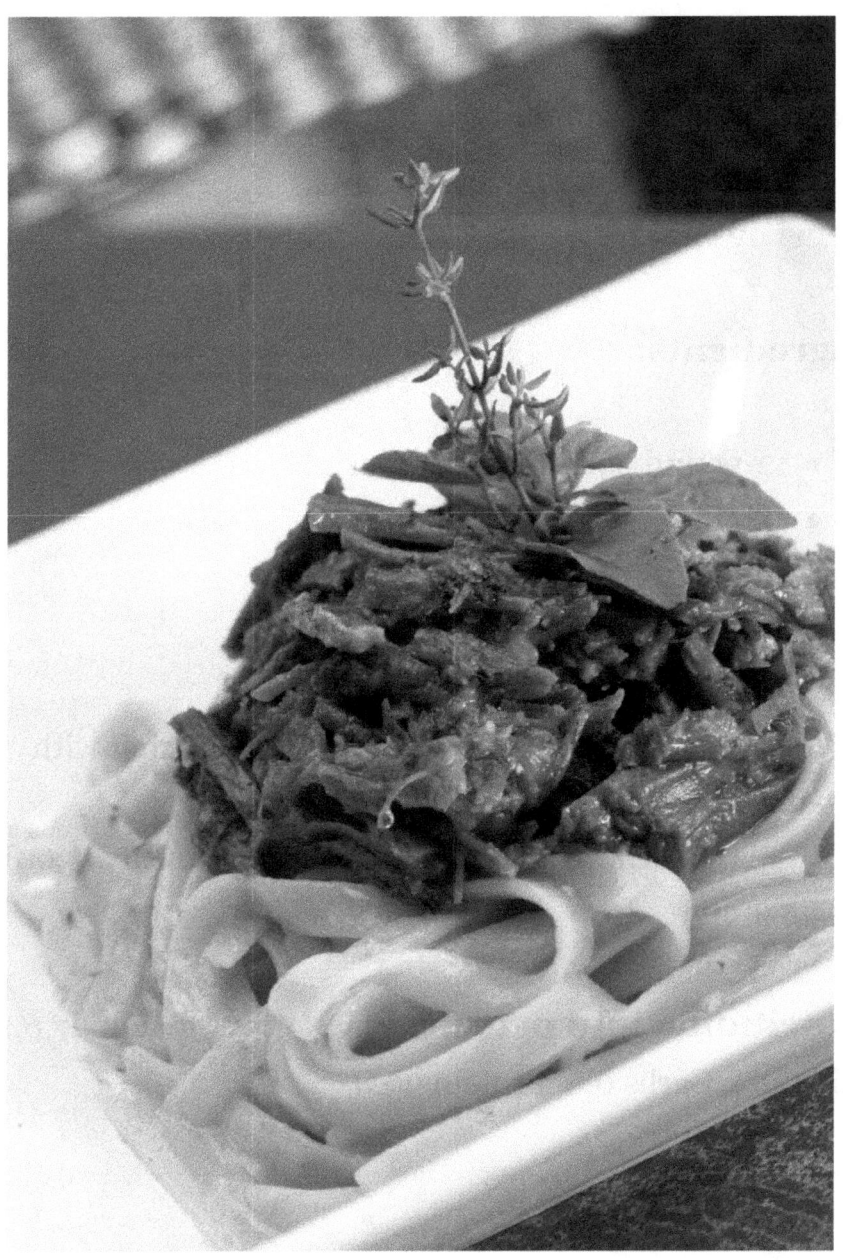

Smoked Paprika Pork

Prep time: 10 minutes
Cook time: 45 minutes
Servings: 6

Ingredients:

- 2-pound pork butt shoulder
- 1 tablespoon smoked paprika
- 1 tablespoon sesame oil

Method:

1. Rub the pork with smoked paprika and brush it with sesame oil.
2. Wrap the meat in the foil and bake in the oven at 360F for 45 minutes.

Nutritional info per serve: Calories 419, Fat 27.6, Fiber 0.4, Carbs 0.6, Protein 39.8

Sweet Pork Belly

Prep time: 10 minutes
Cook time: 50 minutes
Servings: 4

Ingredients:

- 10 oz pork belly
- 1 tablespoon Erythritol
- 1 tablespoon butter
- 1 teaspoon chili powder

Method:

1. Melt the butter in the skillet.
2. Add pork belly and cook it for 4 minutes per side on high heat.
3. Then sprinkle the pork belly with Erythritol and chili powder and bake it in the oven at 360F for 40 minutes.

Nutritional info per serve: Calories 355, Fat 22.1, Fiber 0.2, Carbs 0.4, Protein 32.8

Dill Beef Patties

Prep time: 10 minutes
Cook time: 10 minutes
Servings: 6

Ingredients:

- 1 teaspoon ground coriander
- 1 teaspoon dried dill
- 1 teaspoon onion powder
- 2 cups ground beef
- 3 eggs, beaten
- 1 tablespoon coconut oil

Method:
1. Melt the coconut oil in the skillet.
2. Meanwhile, mix all remaining ingredients in the mixing bowl.
3. Make the patties with the help of the fingertips and put them in the hot coconut oil.
4. Roast the patties for 4 minutes per side on the medium heat.

Nutritional info per serve: Calories 152, Fat 8.4, Fiber 0, Carbs 0.6, Protein 17.8

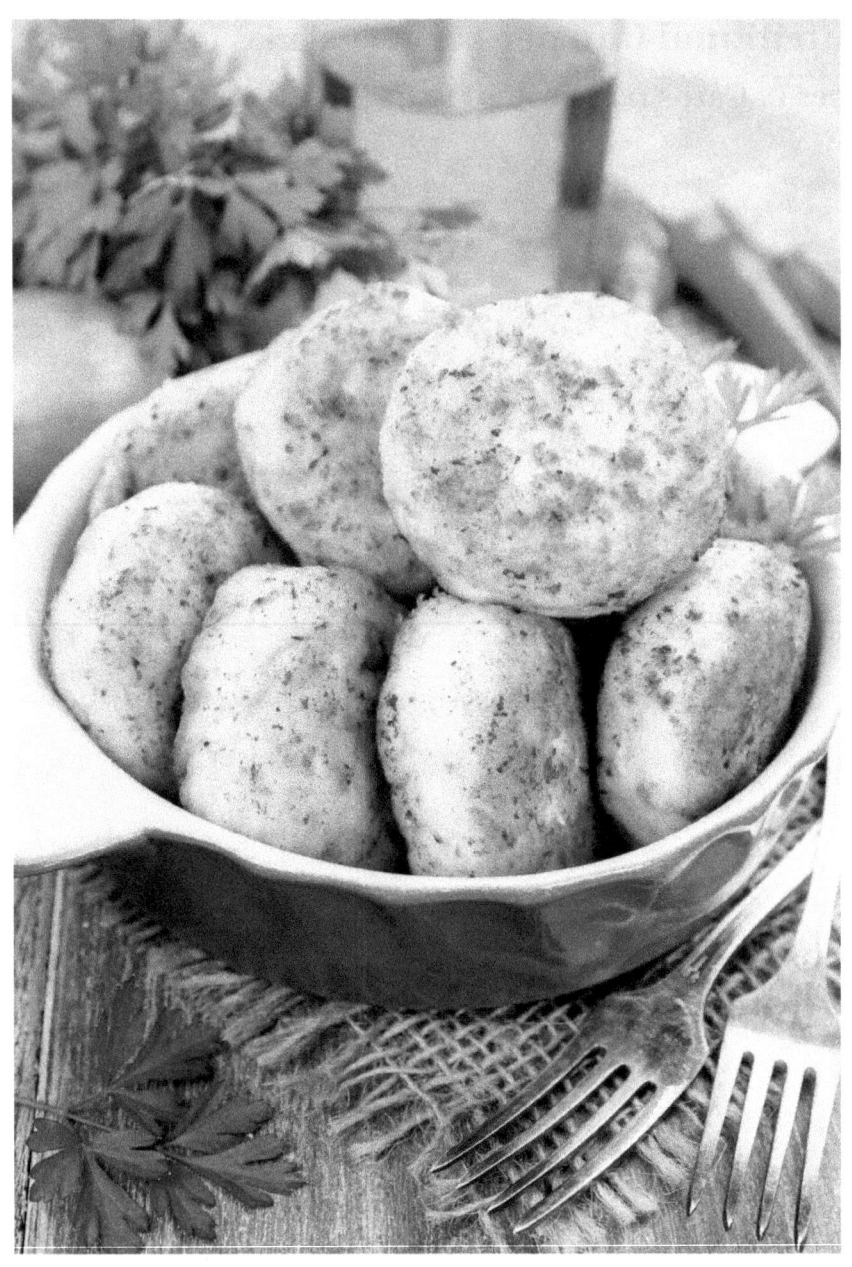

Beef Saute

Prep time: 15 minutes
Cook time: 60 minutes
Servings: 4

Ingredients:

- 1 cup white cabbage, shredded
- 2 cups of water
- 1 teaspoon keto tomato paste
- 1 teaspoon cayenne pepper
- 1 teaspoon ground nutmeg
- 1-pound beef tenderloin, chopped
- 1 tablespoon coconut oil

Method:
1. Melt the coconut oil in the saucepan.
2. Add chopped beef and roast it for 5 minutes. Stir it well.
3. Then add all remaining ingredients and carefully mix.
4. Close the lid and cook the saute on medium-low heat for 55 minutes.

Nutritional info per serve: Calories 273, Fat 14.1, Fiber 0.7, Carbs 1.8, Protein 33.2

Beef and Broccoli Stew

Prep time: 10 minutes
Cook time: 55 minutes
Servings: 5

Ingredients:

- 2 cups broccoli, chopped
- 1-pound beef tenderloin, chopped
- 2 cups chicken broth
- 2 garlic cloves, peeled
- 1 teaspoon ground cinnamon
- 1 tablespoon sesame oil

Method:

1. Roast the beef tenderloin in the saucepan with sesame oil for 2 minutes per side.
2. Then add all remaining ingredients and carefully mix.
3. Close the lid and simmer the stew on medium-low heat for 50 minutes.

Nutritional info per serve: Calories 242, Fat 11.7, Fiber 1.3, Carbs 3.6, Protein 29.3

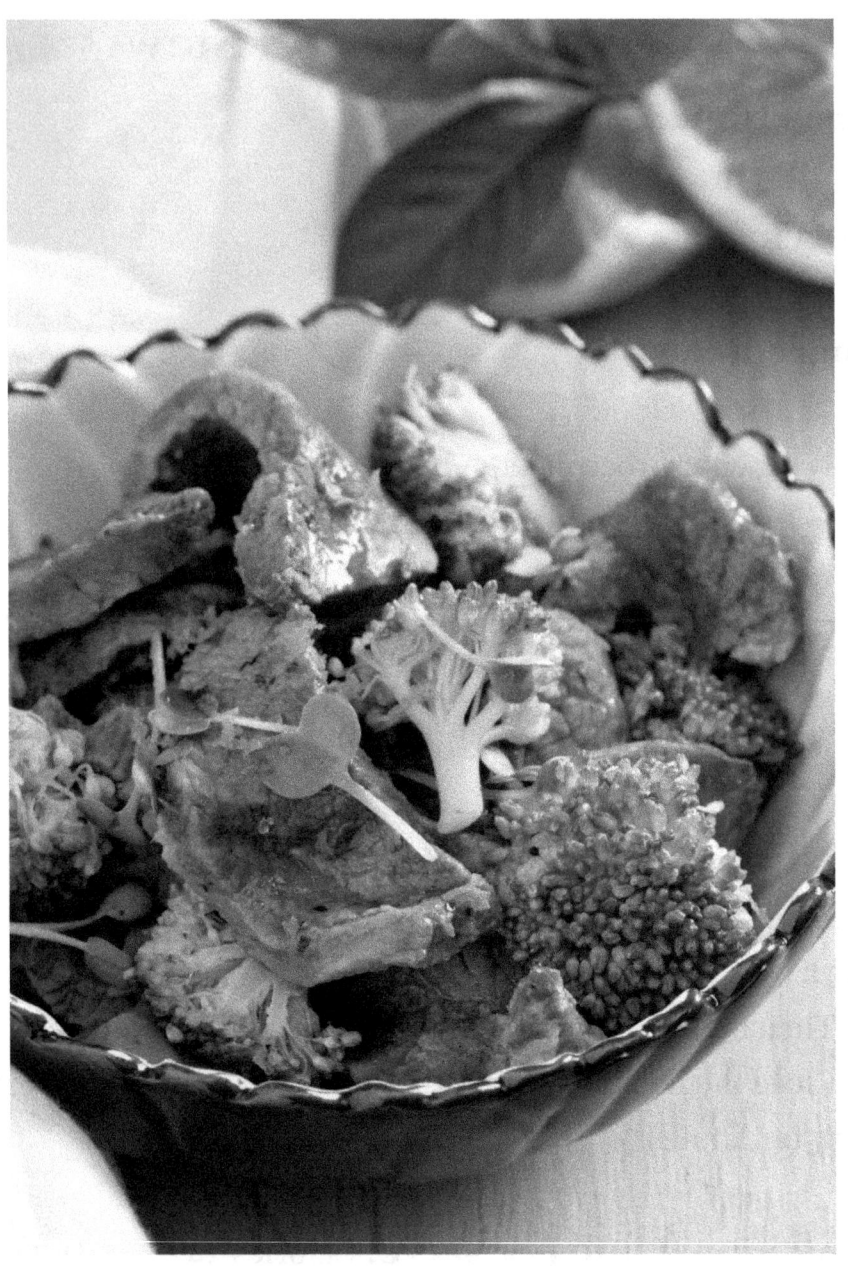

Cinnamon Beef Stew

Prep time: 10 minutes
Cook time: 50 minutes
Servings: 3

Ingredients:

- 8 oz beef fillet, chopped
- 1 teaspoon ground cinnamon
- 1 teaspoon chili powder
- ½ cup of coconut milk
- 1 teaspoon ground paprika
- 1 cup radish, chopped
- 1 cup of water

Method:
1. Put all ingredients in the saucepan and carefully mix.
2. Close the lid and cook the stew on medium heat for 50 minutes.

Nutritional info per serve: Calories 189, Fat 13.2, Fiber 2.5, Carbs 6.4, Protein 13.6

Beef and Eggplant Stew

Prep time: 15 minutes
Cook time: 45 minutes
Servings: 4

Ingredients:

- 1 eggplant, chopped
- 3 spring onions, chopped
- 1-pound beef loin, chopped
- 1 teaspoon keto tomato paste
- 1 teaspoon chili flakes
- 2 cups of water
- 1 teaspoon sesame oil

Method:
1. Preheat the sesame oil in the saucepan and add eggplant.
2. Roast it for 2 minutes per side and add spring onion and beef loin.
3. Stir the mixture and cook it for 6 minutes.
4. Add chili flakes, keto tomato paste, and water. Carefully mix the stew and close the lid.
5. Cook the stew on medium heat for 35 minutes.

Nutritional info per serve: Calories 220, Fat 9.5, Fiber 4.7, Carbs 10.9, Protein 22.4

Beef Rolls

Prep time: 15 minutes
Cook time: 50 minutes
Servings: 6

Ingredients:

- 1-pound beef loin
- 2 oz bacon, sliced
- 1 teaspoon cream cheese
- 1 teaspoon dried parsley
- 2 oz mozzarella, sliced
- ½ cup of water

Method:

1. Beat the beef loin with the help of the kitchen hammer to get the flat fillet.
2. Then rub the meat with dried parsley.
3. Mix cream cheese with mozzarella and put this mixture over the meat.
4. Roll the meat into a roll and wrap in the bacon.
5. Secure the meat roll with the toothpicks if needed and put in the baking pan.

6. Add water and cook the meal in the oven at 360F for 50 minutes.

Nutritional info per serve: Calories 217, Fat 12.1, Fiber 0, Carbs 0.5, Protein 26.4

Mint Lamb Chops

Prep time: 10 minutes
Cook time: 10 minutes
Servings: 4

Ingredients:

- 1 teaspoon dried mint
- 4 lamb chops
- ½ teaspoon salt
- 1 tablespoon avocado oil

Method:
1. Preheat the avocado oil well.
2. Rub the lamb chops with dried mint and salt.
3. Then put the meat in the hot oil and roast them for 5 minutes per side on the medium heat.

Nutritional info per serve: Calories 163, Fat 6.7, Fiber 0.2, Carbs 0.2, Protein 23.9

Chipotle Lamb Ribs

Prep time: 15 minutes
Cook time: 20 minutes
Servings: 6

Ingredients:

- 2-pound lamb ribs
- 1 tablespoon chipotle pepper, minced
- 2 tablespoons sesame oil
- 1 teaspoon apple cider vinegar

Method:

1. Mix lamb ribs with all ingredients and leave to marinate for 10 minutes.
2. Then transfer the lamb ribs and all marinade in the baking tray and cook the meat in the oven at 360F for 40 minutes. Flip the ribs on another side after 20 minutes of cooking.

Nutritional info per serve: Calories 392, Fat 24.7, Fiber 0, Carbs 0.2, Protein 39.6

Lamb and Pecan Salad

Prep time: 10 minutes
Cook time: 10 minutes
Servings: 4

Ingredients:

- 2 lamb chops
- 1 tablespoon sesame oil
- 2 pecans, chopped
- 2 cups lettuce, chopped
- 1 teaspoon cayenne pepper
- 1 tablespoon avocado oil

Method:
1. Sprinkle the lamb chops with cayenne pepper and put in the hot skillet.
2. Add sesame oil and roast the meat for 4 minutes per side.
3. Then chop the lamb chops and put them in the salad bowl.
4. Add all remaining ingredients and carefully mix the salad.

Nutritional info per serve: Calories 168, Fat 12.1, Fiber 1., Carbs 2.3, Protein 12.9

Lime Ribs

Prep time: 10 minutes
Cook time: 10 minutes
Servings: 6

Ingredients:

- 3-pounds pork ribs, chopped
- 2 tablespoons lime juice
- 1 teaspoon lime zest, grated
- 2 tablespoons sesame seeds
- ½ teaspoon salt
- ½ teaspoon ground black pepper

Method:

1. In the shallow bowl, mix lime juice, lime zest, sesame seeds, salt, and ground black pepper.
2. Mix the pork ribs with lime juice mixture and grill in the preheated to 390F grill for 5 minutes per side.

Nutritional info per serve: Calories 638, Fat 41.7, Fiber 0.5, Carbs 1.2, Protein 60.6

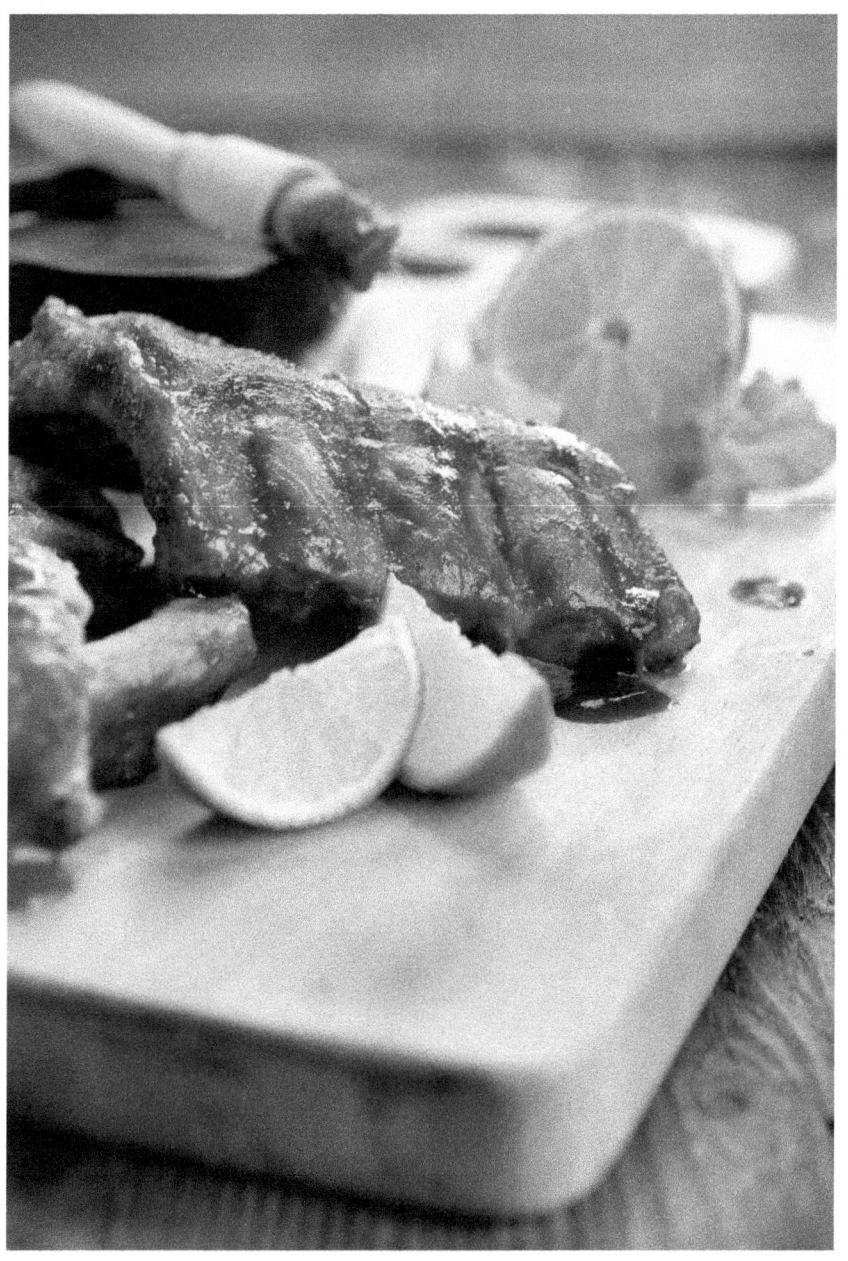

Notes

www.ingramcontent.com/pod-product-compliance
Lightning Source LLC
Chambersburg PA
CBHW070723030426
42336CB00013B/1905